Paramedic Care
Principles & Practice
Patient Assessment

Workbook
Fourth Edition

Paramedic Care
Principles & Practice
Patient Assessment

Workbook
Fourth Edition

ROBERT S. PORTER

REVISED BY

MELISSA ALEXANDER, Ed. D., NREMT-P
Lake Superior State University
Sault Sainte Marie, Michigan

BRYAN E. BLEDSOE, DO, FACEP, FAAEM, EMT-P
Professor of Emergency Medicine
Director, Prehospital and Disaster Medicine Fellowship
University of Nevada School of Medicine
Attending Emergency Physician
University Medical Center of Southern Nevada
Medical Director, MedicWest Ambulance
Las Vegas, Nevada

ROBERT S. PORTER, MA, EMT-P
Senior Advanced Life Support Educator
Madison County Emergency Medical Services
Canastota, New York

RICHARD A. CHERRY, MS, NREMT-P
Director of Training
Northern Onondaga Volunteer Ambulance
Liverpool, New York

PEARSON

Boston Columbus Indianapolis New York San Francisco Upper Saddle River
Amsterdam Cape Town Dubai London Madrid Milan Munich Paris Montréal Toronto
Delhi Mexico City São Paulo Sydney Hong Kong Seoul Singapore Taipei Tokyo

Publisher: *Julie Levin Alexander*
Publisher's Assistant: *Regina Bruno*
Editor-in-Chief: *Marlene McHugh Pratt*
Senior Managing Editor for Development: *Lois Berlowitz*
Editorial Project Manager: *Triple SSS Press Media
    Development, Inc.*
Assistant Editor: *Jonathan Cheung*
Director of Marketing: *David Gesell*
Marketing Manager: *Brian Hoehl*
Marketing Specialist: *Michael Sirinides*
Managing Editor for Production: *Patrick Walsh*
Production Liaison: *Faye Gemmellaro*
Production Editor: *Muralidharan Krishnamurthy/S4Carlisle
    Publishing Services*
Manufacturing Manager: *Ilene Sanford*
Cover Design: *Kathryn Foot*
Cover Image: *© corepics/Shutterstock*
Composition: *S4Carlisle Publishing Services*
Cover and Interior Printer/Binder: *Edwards Brothers*

NOTICE ON CPR AND ECC

The national standards for cardiopulmonary resuscitation (CPR) and emergency cardiovascular care (ECC) are reviewed and revised on a regular basis and may change slightly after this manual is printed. It is important that you know the most current procedures for CPR and ECC, both for the classroom and your patients. The most current information may always be downloaded from www.bradybooks.com or obtained from the appropriate credentialing agency.

NOTICE ON CARE PROCEDURES

It is the intent of the authors and publisher that this Workbook be used as part of a formal Paramedic program taught by qualified instructors and supervised by a licensed physician. The procedures described in this Workbook are based upon consultation with EMS and medical authorities. The authors and publisher have taken care to make certain that these procedures reflect currently accepted clinical practice; however, they cannot be considered absolute recommendations.

The material in this Workbook contains the most current information available at the time of publication. However, federal, state, and local guidelines concerning clinical practices, including, without limitation, those governing infection control and universal precautions, change rapidly. The reader should note, therefore, that the new regulations may require changes in some procedures.

It is the responsibility of the reader to familiarize himself or herself with the policies and procedures set by federal, state, and local agencies as well as the institution or agency where the reader is employed. The authors and the publisher of this Workbook disclaim any liability, loss, or risk resulting directly or indirectly from the suggested procedures and theory, from any undetected errors, or from the reader's misunderstanding of the text. It is the reader's responsibility to stay informed of any new changes or recommendations made by any federal, state, and local agency as well as by his or her employing institution or agency.

Brady
is an imprint of

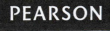

www.bradybooks.com

10 9 8 7 6 5 4 3 2 1
ISBN 10: 0-13-211107-1
ISBN 13: 978-0-13-211107-2

Dedication

This workbook is dedicated to the important people in your life: your wife/husband, mother, father, sister, brother . . . and friends who support you and the time and passion you devote to Emergency Medical Service.
Without them, this endeavor would be lonely and much less rewarding.

–ROBERT S. PORTER

CONTENTS

INTRODUCTION

Welcome to the self-instructional Workbook for *Paramedic Care: Principles & Practice*. This Workbook is designed to help guide you through an educational program for initial or refresher training that follows the guidelines of the 2009 *National EMS Education Standards*. The Workbook is designed to be used either in conjunction with your instructor or as a self-study guide you use on your own.

This Workbook features many different ways to help you learn the material necessary to become a paramedic, as described next.

Features

Review of Chapter Objectives

Each chapter of *Paramedic Care: Principles & Practice* begins with objectives that identify the important information and principles addressed in the chapter reading. To help you identify and learn this material, each Workbook chapter reviews the important content elements addressed by these objectives as presented in the text.

Case Study Review

Each chapter of *Paramedic Care: Principles & Practice* includes a case study, introducing and highlighting important principles presented in the chapter. The Workbook reviews these case studies and points out much of the essential information and many of the applied principles they describe.

Content Self-Evaluation

Each chapter of *Paramedic Care: Principles & Practice* presents an extensive narrative explanation of the principles of paramedic practice. The Workbook chapter (or chapter section) contains between 10 and 50 multiple-choice questions to test your reading comprehension of the textbook material and to give you experience taking typical emergency medical service examinations.

Special Projects

The Workbook contains several projects that are special learning experiences designed to help you remember the information and principles necessary to perform as a paramedic. Special projects include crossword puzzle, fill-in-the-blank exercises, and a variety of other activities.

Personal Benchmarking

The Workbook provides several exercises that direct you to evaluate elements of the patient assessment process on yourself. These exercises help you develop your assessment skills and use normal findings as benchmarks for reference when you begin your career as a paramedic.

Content Review

The Workbook provides a comprehensive review of the material presented in Volume 3 of *Paramedic Care: Principles & Practice*. After the last text chapter has been covered, the Workbook presents an extensive content self-evaluation component that helps you recall and build upon the knowledge you have gained by reading the text, attending class, and completing the earlier Workbook chapters.

Patient Scenario Flash Cards

At the end of this Workbook are scenario flash cards, which are designed to help you practice the processes of investigating both the chief complaint and the past medical history. Each card contains the dispatch information and results of the scene size-up and then prompts you to inquire into either the patient's major symptoms or past medical history.

HOW TO USE THIS SELF-INSTRUCTIONAL WORKBOOK

The self-instructional Workbook accompanying *Paramedic Care: Principles & Practice* may be used as directed by your instructor or independently by you during your course of instruction. The following recommendations are intended to guide you in using the Workbook independently.

- Examine your course schedule and identify the appropriate text chapter or other assigned reading.

- Read the assigned chapter in *Paramedic Care: Principles & Practice* carefully. Do this in a relaxed environment, free of distractions, and give yourself adequate time to read and digest the material. The information presented in *Paramedic Care: Principles & Practice* is often technically complex and demanding, but it is very important that you comprehend it. Be sure that you read the chapter carefully enough to understand and remember what you have read.

- Carefully read the Review of Chapter Objectives at the beginning of each Workbook chapter (or section). This material includes both the objectives listed in *Paramedic Care: Principles & Practice* and narrative descriptions of their content. If you do not understand or remember what is discussed from your reading, refer to the referenced pages and reread them carefully. If you still do not feel comfortable with your understanding of any objective, consider asking your instructor about it.

- Reread the case study in *Paramedic Care: Principles & Practice*, and then read the Case Study Review in the Workbook. Note the important points regarding assessment and care that the Case Study Review highlights and be sure that you understand and agree with the analysis of the call. If you have any questions or concerns, ask your instructor to clarify the information.

- Take the Content Self-Evaluation at the end of each Workbook chapter (or section), answering each question carefully. Do this in a quiet environment, free from distractions, and allow yourself adequate time to complete the exercise. Correct your self-evaluation by consulting the answers at the back of the Workbook, and determine the percentage you have answered correctly (the number you got right divided by the total number of questions). If you have answered most of the questions correctly (85 to 90 percent), review those that you missed by rereading the material on the pages listed in the answer key and be sure you understand which answer is correct and why. If you have more than a few questions wrong (less than 85 percent correct), look for incorrect answers that are grouped together. This suggests that you did not understand a particular topic in the reading. Reread the text dealing with that topic carefully, and then retest yourself on the questions you got wrong. If incorrect answers are spread throughout the chapter content, reread the chapter and retake the Content Self-Evaluation to ensure that you understand the material. If you don't understand why your answer to a question is incorrect after reviewing the text, consult with your instructor.

- In a similar fashion, complete the exercises in the Special Projects section of the Workbook chapters (or sections). These exercises are specifically designed to help you learn and remember the essential principles and information presented in *Paramedic Care: Principles & Practice*.

- When you have completed this volume of *Paramedic Care: Principles & Practice* and its accompanying Workbook, prepare for a course test by reviewing both the text in its entirety and your class notes. Then take the Content Review examination in the Workbook. Again, review your score and any questions you have answered incorrectly by referring to the text and rereading the page or pages where the material is presented. If you note groupings of wrong answers, review the entire range of pages or the full chapter they represent.

If, during your completion of the Workbook exercises, you have any questions that either the textbook or Workbook doesn't answer, write them down and ask your instructor about them. Prehospital emergency medicine is a complex and complicated subject, and answers are not always black and white. It is also common for different EMS systems to use differing methods of care. The questions you bring up in class, and your instructor's answers to them, will help you expand and complete your knowledge of prehospital emergency medical care.

GUIDELINES TO BETTER TEST-TAKING

The knowledge you will gain from reading the textbook, completing the exercises in the Workbook, listening in your paramedic class, and participating in your clinical and field experience will prepare you to care for patients who are seriously ill or injured. However, before you can practice these skills, you will have to pass several classroom written exams and your state's certification exam. Your performance on these exams will depend not only on your knowledge but also on your ability to answer test questions correctly. The following guidelines are designed to help your performance on tests and to better demonstrate your knowledge of pre-hospital emergency care.

1. Relax and be calm during the test.

A test is designed to measure what you have learned and to tell you and your instructor how well you are doing. An exam is not designed to intimidate or punish you. Consider it a challenge, and just try to do your best. Get plenty of sleep before the examination. Avoid coffee or other stimulants for a few hours before the exam, and be prepared.

Reread the text chapters, review the objectives in the Workbook, and review your class notes. It might be helpful to work with one or two other students and ask each other questions. This type of practice helps everyone better understand the knowledge presented in your course of study.

2. Read the questions carefully.

Read each word of the question and all the answers slowly. Words such as "except" or "not" may change the entire meaning of the question. If you miss such words, you may answer the question incorrectly even though you know the right answer.

Example:
The art and science of emergency medical services involves all of the following EXCEPT

    A. sincerity and compassion.
    B. respect for human dignity.
    C. placing patient care before personal safety.
    D. delivery of sophisticated emergency medical care.
    E. none of the above.

The correct answer is C, unless you miss the "EXCEPT."

3. Read each answer carefully.

Read each and every answer carefully. Although the first answer may be absolutely correct, so may the rest, and thus the best answer might be "all of the above."

Example:
Indirect medical direction is considered to be

    A. treatment protocols.
    B. training and education.
    C. quality assurance.
    D. chart review.
    E. all of the above.

Although answers A, B, C, and D are each correct, the best and only acceptable answer is "all of the above," E.

4. Delay answering questions you don't understand and look for clues.

When a question seems confusing or you don't know the answer, note it on your answer sheet and come back to it later. This will ensure that you have time to complete the test. You will also find that other questions on the test may give you hints to answer the one you've skipped over. It will also prevent you from being frustrated with an early question and letting it affect your performance.

Example:

Upon successful completion of a course of training as an EMT-P, most states will

    A. certify you. (correct)
    B. license you.
    C. register you.
    D. recognize you as a paramedic.
    E. issue you a permit.

Another question, later in the exam, may suggest the right answer:

The action of one state in recognizing the certification of another is called

    A. reciprocity. (correct)
    B. national registration.
    C. licensure.
    D. registration.
    E. extended practice.

5. Answer all questions.

Even if you do not know the right answer, do not leave a question blank. A blank question is always wrong, whereas a guess might be correct. If you can eliminate some of the answers as wrong, do so. It will increase the chances of a correct guess.

A multiple-choice question with five answers gives a 20 percent chance of a correct guess. If you can eliminate one or more incorrect answers, you increase your odds of a correct guess to 25 percent, 33 percent, and so on. An unanswered question has a 0 percent chance of being correct.

Just before turning in your answer sheet, check to be sure that you have not left any items blank.

Example:

When a paramedic is called by the patient (through the dispatcher) to the scene of a medical emergency, the medical direction physician has established a physician/patient relationship.

    A. True
    B. False

A true/false question gives you a 50 percent chance of a correct guess.

The hospital health professional(s) responsible for sorting patients as they arrive at the emergency department is/are usually the

    A. emergency physician.
    B. ward clerk.
    C. emergency nurse.
    D. trauma surgeon.
    E. both A and C. (correct)

Paramedic Care
Principles & Practice
Patient Assessment

Workbook

Fourth Edition

Chapter

1

Scene Size-Up

Review of Chapter Objectives

With each chapter of the Workbook, we identify the objectives and the important elements of the text content. You should review these items and refer to the pages listed if any points are not clear.

After reading this chapter, you should be able to:

1. **Define key terms introduced in this chapter.**

   Knowing and being able to apply the key terms in each chapter is critical to understanding chapter concepts. Write the list of key terms. Then write the definition of each one in your own words. Check your understanding by confirming the definitions in the text glossary. Correct any misunderstandings. Create a study aid by writing each key term on the front of an index card and the definition on the back. Use the cards to quiz yourself, or to have someone quiz you.

2. **Place the components of scene size-up in the overall context of an emergency call.** pp. 2–4

   Scene size-up is the essential first stage of every emergency call. It is not a step-by-step process, but a series of timely decisions you will make to ensure that you and your crew remain safe, and secure the necessary resources to manage the scene and care for the patient. The components of scene size-up are presented in order in the text, but you will make critical decisions about the scene in the order that the unique features of each scene dictate. Not only is scene size-up your initial step when approaching the scene, but it is an on-going process. Scenes are dynamic and can change quickly.

3. **Describe the scope and purposes of scene size-up.** pp. 2–4

   The scope and purposes of the scene size up includes answering the following critical decisions:

   - Is the scene safe to enter?
   - Which standard infection control precautions will be appropriate?
   - What additional resources will be necessary?
   - Have we located all of the patients?
   - What does the mechanism of injury or nature of illness suggest?

   Revisit these decisions throughout the call, as situations can always change.

4. **Given a variety of scenarios, make observations of the scene to do the following:**

   Identify indications of potential hazards pp. 6–12
   Scene safety means doing everything possible to ensure a safe environment for yourself, your crew, other responding personnel, your patient, and any bystanders. If a scene is not safe, you must not enter it until it is made safe. You must take actions to make the scene safe, if possible, or request the specialized resources needed to make the scene safe. Among the hazards you must look for are environmental

hazards, such as weather, terrain, and water, as well as other hazards such as electricity, confined spaces, hazardous materials, violence, and hazards associated with roadway rescue operations.

Determine the mechanism of injury or nature of the illness pp. 15–16
Mechanism of injury is the combined strength, direction, and nature of forces that injure a patient. By carefully evaluating a trauma scene, you can anticipate the location and seriousness of potential injuries that may not be obvious based on examination of your patient alone. Consider the distance of falls, how the patient landed, and the surface he landed on. Consider the direction and force of impact in vehicle collisions, the location of the patient in the vehicle, and what types of restraints were used. With penetrating injuries, consider the type of weapon used and the force associated with it. The nature of an illness can be determined by questioning bystanders and the patient, paying attention to your patient's position and general appearance, and recognizing clues at the scene, such as medications or oxygen.

Identify all patients involved pp. 13–15
Scene size-up involves searching the area to locate all patients. Determine the total number of patients and the resources needed to assess, manage, and transport them. Vehicle collisions and exposure to toxins, such as carbon monoxide, are some examples of scenes where you must be particularly alert to the possibility of multiple patients.

Identify the need for specific additional resources pp. 12–13
Specific types of scenes require specific special resources. Depending on the situation, you may need heavy duty rescue for extrication, or additional medical personnel, equipment, or supplies. You may need to call upon a hazardous materials team; law enforcement; special rescue crews for rough terrain or water rescue; water, gas, or electric utility personnel; or a variety of other resources. Be careful that you do not overestimate your capabilities for managing a situation; call for resources when they are needed.

Make decisions about Standard Precautions and personal protective equipment pp. 4–5
Decisions about Standard Precautions are based on the initial and evolving characteristics of the call. Important aspects of Standard Precautions include hand hygiene, protective gloves, masks and protective eyewear, HEPA and N-95 respirators, gowns, and disposable resuscitation equipment.

Communicate findings and request resources. pp. 6–16
Once you have identified the characteristics of the scene, request the needed resources, such as rescue teams, additional ambulances, law enforcement, and utility company personnel. Do not overestimate your ability to manage a scene.

5. **When confronted with a variety of potential hazards in a scenario, take actions that protect your safety and the safety of your crew, the patient, bystanders, and the public.** pp. 6–16

Your first responsibility is for your own safety, and that of your crew. If a scene is not safe, do not enter it until it is made safe. If necessary, request the specialized resources needed to address specific hazards. Protect your patient from hazards, and keep bystanders away from hazards at the scene.

Case Study Review

It is important to review each emergency response you participate in as a paramedic. Similarly, we will review the case study that precedes each chapter. We will address the important points of the response as addressed by the chapter. Often, this will include scene size-up, patient assessment, patient management, patient packaging, and transport.

Reread the case study on page 2 in Paramedic Care: Patient Assessment. *This case study draws attention to the value of taking time to observe the scene as you approach, rather than rushing in.*

Dean and Kyle have responded to a call for a person slumped over the steering wheel of a vehicle. Kyle's lack of experience makes him less cautious about safety than his more experienced partner, Dean. Dean observes several indications of danger as they approach the scene and stops Kyle from rushing up to a potentially dangerous situation. Dean points out the clues that he sees to Kyle, and then, because they suspect hazardous materials, he parks the ambulance upwind from the scene and advises dispatch so they can notify the appropriate resources to respond. Kyle and Dean take measures to keep bystanders and the public safe by blocking off the area, and advise incoming personnel of the dangers. This case study reinforces the fact that nothing is more important than rescuer safety.

Content Self-Evaluation

Each chapter in this Workbook includes a short content review. The questions are designed to test your ability to remember what you have read. At the end of this Workbook, you can find the answers to the questions, as well as the pages where the topic of each question is discussed in the text. If you answer the question incorrectly or are unsure of the answer, review the pages listed.

MULTIPLE CHOICE

_____ 1. After the initial scene size-up, if necessary, you should inform the dispatcher of
   A. the nature of the medical or trauma emergency.
   B. what resources you need.
   C. general impression.
   D. what actions you and your crew are taking.
   E. all of the above except C.

_____ 2. Which of the following is NOT a component of the scene size-up?
   A. Consideration of c-spine
   B. Making patient transport decisions
   C. Location of all patients
   D. Analysis of mechanism of injury/nature of the illness
   E. Scene safety

_____ 3. Which of the following Standard Precautions devices will you employ with every patient you treat?
   A. Latex or vinyl gloves   D. Gown
   B. Protective eyewear   E. Both B and C
   C. Face mask

_____ 4. Whenever you plan to intubate a patient, you should wear
   A. latex or vinyl gloves and a gown.
   B. protective eyewear, a gown, and a face mask.
   C. latex or vinyl gloves, protective eyewear, and a face mask.
   D. protective eyewear and a gown.
   E. latex or vinyl gloves.

_____ 5. The HEPA respirator is designed to filter out which of the following pathogens that may be encountered when providing prehospital emergency care?
   A. Tuberculosis   D. Flu
   B. Smallpox   E. Tetanus toxoid
   C. Anthrax

_____ 6. The intent of the safety analysis portion of the scene survey is to ensure the safety of
   A. the patient.   D. yourself.
   B. bystanders.   E. all of the above.
   C. fellow responders.

_____ 7. To handle a scene safety issue properly, you must be
   A. properly trained.
   B. properly equipped.
   C. properly clothed.
   D. prepared to attempt rescue procedures in which you have not been trained.
   E. A, B, and C.

_____ 8. Potential hazards to rule out before entering the scene include all of the following EXCEPT
   A. fire.
   B. electrocution.
   C. whether the patient is bleeding.
   D. structural collapse.
   E. broken glass and jagged metal.

_____ 9. When called to a shooting or domestic disturbance, until the police arrive and secure the scene you should remain
   A. a few blocks away.
   B. outside the residence.
   C. just down the street.
   D. at the door but do not enter.
   E. within direct line of sight from the scene.

_____ 10. At which of the following incidents would you LEAST expect to discover more than one patient in your scene size-up?
   A. A two-car collision
   B. A carbon monoxide poisoning in a home
   C. A car crash in which a child seat and diaper bag are visible
   D. A fall out of a tree
   E. A hazardous materials spill in a high school chemistry lab

_____ 11. You should delay the call for additional ambulances until you begin your primary assessment because you will not have enough information to determine the needs of the scene until then.
   A. True
   B. False

_____ 12. The two important functions that must begin immediately in a mass-casualty situation are
   A. triage and incident management.
   B. rescue and triage.
   C. firefighting and rescue.
   D. incident management and extrication.
   E. incident management and scene isolation.

_____ 13. The responsibilities of the triage person at the disaster scene include all of the following EXCEPT
   A. determining a patient's priority for immediate transport.
   B. determining a patient's priority for delayed transport.
   C. performing simple but lifesaving procedures.
   D. providing intensive care on salvageable patients.
   E. identifying patients who will not be treated or transported.

_____ 14. The analysis of mechanism of injury examines
   A. body locations affected.
   B. strength of the crash forces.
   C. direction of the crash forces.
   D. nature of the crash forces.
   E. all of the above.

_____ 15. The index of suspicion is best defined as
   A. patient priority for care based on the MOI.
   B. anticipation of the nature of forces involved in an accident.
   C. prediction of injuries based on the MOI.
   D. prediction of degree of injury based on the patient's appearance.
   E. none of the above.

_____ **16.** The nature of the illness is determined from information you receive from

    A. the patient.
    D. scene clues.
    B. the patient's family.
    E. all of the above.
    C. bystanders.

MATCHING

Write the letter of the protective equipment in the space provided next to the appropriate reason for its use.

  A. disposable gloves

  B. mask and protective eyewear

  C. HEPA or N-95 respirator

  D. gown

  E. disposable resuscitation equipment

  F. hand hygiene

_____ **17.** Worn to protect the face when performing airway procedures or when blood spatter is likely

_____ **18.** Before and after all patient contact

_____ **19.** Used to protect your clothing from blood splashes

_____ **20.** Worn for all patient contact; changed between patients

_____ **21.** Design for single-patient use to prevent spread of infection from one patient to another

_____ **22.** Worn when in contact with a patient with confirmed or suspected TB, influenza, or meningitis

SHORT ANSWER

23. What are the characteristics of a confined space, as defined by OSHA?

    A. _____

    B. _____

    C. _____

    D. _____

24. Give examples of each type of hazardous material listed below.

    A. Chemical _____

    B. Biological _____

    C. Radiologic _____

    D. Explosive _____

25. List the four "don'ts" of approaching a potential hazardous materials scene.

    A. _____

    B. _____

    C. _____

    D. _____

Special Project

Scene Size-Up Exercise

Review the accompanying photographs and identify the likely hazards you should suspect at each scene.

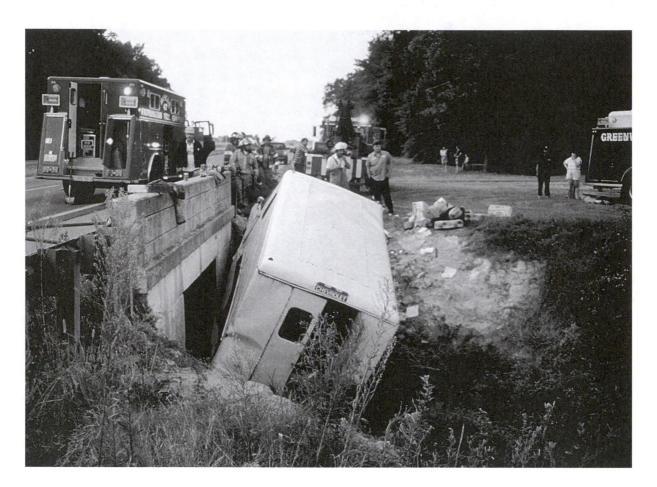

A. _____

_____

_____

_____

_____

_____

_____

_____

_____

_____

_____

_____

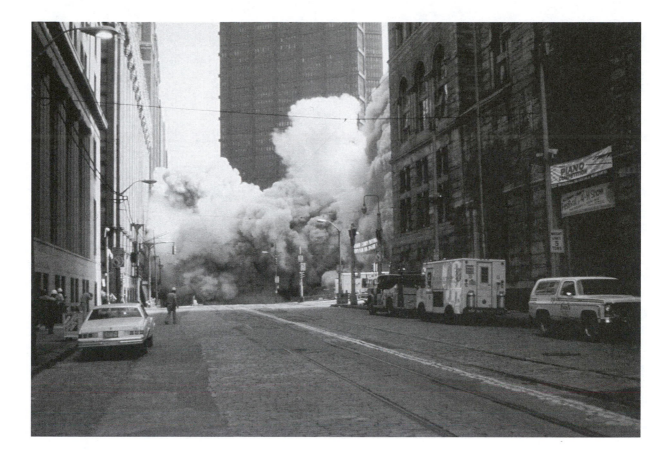

B. _____
_____
_____
_____
_____
_____
_____
_____
_____
_____
_____
_____
_____
_____
_____

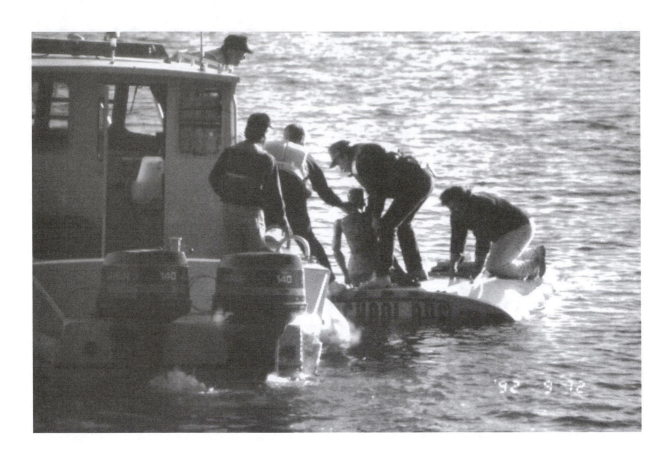

C. _____
_____
_____
_____
_____
_____
_____
_____
_____
_____
_____
_____
_____
_____

©2013 Pearson Education, Inc.
Paramedic Care: Principles & Practice, Vol. 3, 4th Ed.

Primary Assessment

Review of Chapter Objectives

After reading this chapter, you should be able to:

1. **Define key terms introduced in this chapter.**

   Knowing and being able to apply the key terms in each chapter is critical to understanding chapter concepts. Write the list of key terms. Then write the definition of each one in your own words. Check your understanding by confirming the definitions in the text glossary. Correct any misunderstandings. Create a study aid by writing each key term on the front of an index card and the definition on the back. Use the cards to quiz yourself, or to have someone quiz you.

2. **Behave in ways that demonstrate empathy and compassion in your interactions with patients.** pp. 21–22

   Patients expect you to be nice to them, and to treat them the way you would want your family to be treated. Focus on the patient and explain things. Reassure patients and do not trivialize their concerns.

3. **Respond appropriately to patients' concerns and complaints.** pp. 22

   Listen to your patient and gather as many clues as possible. Establish rapport and let the patient know you take his concerns seriously, even as you provide reassurance.

4. **Place the primary assessment in the overall context of an emergency call.** pp. 21

   The primary assessment is the basis for all emergency medical care. As soon as you have completed a scene size-up and established the safety of the scene, you perform a primary assessment. During the primary assessment you look for immediately life-threatening problems with the airway, breathing, and circulation and intervene to correct them. Steps of the primary assessment include forming a general impression, stabilizing the cervical spine as needed, assessing a baseline mental status, assessing and managing the airway, assessing and managing breathing, assessing and managing circulation, and determining priorities of care and transport. After correcting immediate life threats, you make decisions regarding how quickly to prepare for transport and what treatment should be carried out at the scene. The primary assessment, from beginning to end, should take less than 1 minute, unless interventions are needed. The primary assessment is repeated as part of patient reassessment.

5. **Given a variety of scenarios, identify conditions of the airway, breathing, and circulation that present an immediate threat to life.** pp. 21–29

   As with the scene size-up, think of the primary assessment not as a step-by-step process, but as a series of critical decisions based on what you find. In most cases, you will proceed systematically through the

ABCs, but sometimes the situation may determine how much priority you give to any one component. Conditions that require immediate intervention or make the patient a high priority for transport include a decreased level of responsiveness, abnormal or absent breathing, airway compromise or obstruction, pulselessness, hemorrhage, and signs of hypoperfusion.

6. **Identify situations in which the approach to a patient is sequenced**
   circulation, airway, breathing. **pp. 21–22**

As part of forming a general impression, you immediately determine whether patient "looks dead" or "doesn't look dead." The approach is different, based on your general impression. For patients who are obviously not dead, that is, patients who are awake, moving, and have indications of circulation and breathing, the order of assessment is *airway, breathing, circulation*. For those patients who "look dead," that is, appear unresponsive and do not appear to have normal breathing, the highest priority becomes determining whether or not the patient has a pulse. For patients who do not have a carotid pulse that can be detected in less than 10 seconds, you begin CPR, starting with 30 chest compressions (as long as there are no contraindications to resuscitation). In cardiac arrest, the highest priority is restoring circulation through chest compressions and, if indicated, defibrillation.

7. **Explain the importance of establishing the patient's baseline condition and performing primary assessment as part of the reassessment process.** **pp. 21–23**

In order to track trends in a patient's condition, you first must establish his baseline condition. Later assessments are compared to the baseline to determine whether the patient is stable, improving, or deteriorating, which allows you to make decisions about his ongoing care and, if necessary, revise his priority status. This information also allows the medical team at the hospital to make decisions about the patient's care when he arrives at the emergency department.

8. **Use scene size-up and primary assessment findings to make decisions about the priorities of patient care and transport.** **p. 29**

If findings of the primary assessment suggest serious illness or injury, that is, any problem with mental status, airway, breathing, or circulation, perform a rapid head-to-toe assessment to identify other life threats and transport the patient immediately to the nearest appropriate facility that can deliver definitive care. Do not delay transport for detailed assessments and procedures that you can provide en route to the hospital.

9. **For a variety of patients, demonstrate each of the steps of primary assessment as follows:**

   a. **Form a general impression** **pp. 21–22**
   Base your first impression on the information you gather from the environment, the mechanism of injury, the nature of the illness, your patient's posture and overall look, the chief complaint, and your instincts. Determine the patient's mechanism of injury or nature of the illness, if there was not enough information in the scene size-up to do so.

   b. **Stabilize the cervical spine, as needed** **p. 22**
   If there is a significant mechanism of injury, provide manual stabilization of the cervical spine. Approximately 2 percent of patients with significant blunt trauma have a cervical spine injury. The risk triples if the patient has severe craniofacial trauma. For children, pad beneath the shoulders to compensate for the large occiput.

   c. **Assess the baseline mental status** **p. 23**
   Initially, determine whether the patient is alert, responds to verbal stimuli, responds to painful stimuli, or is unresponsive (AVPU). In the patient who responds only to pain, note whether there is decerebrate or decorticate posturing. Take steps to protect the airway of a patient with decreased level of responsiveness. The Glasgow Coma Scale uses the information collected during assessment of the baseline mental status to assign a numeric score to the level of responsiveness.

   d. **Assess and manage the airway** **pp. 24–26**
   In a patient who is not awake and not able to speak clearly, you must take additional steps to assess and ensure the patency of the airway. In an unresponsive patient in a supine position, the tongue

©2013 Pearson Education, Inc.
Paramedic Care: Principles & Practice, Vol. 3, 4th Ed.

often obstructs the airway. This is easily remedied using manual airway maneuvers and basic airway adjuncts. Once the airway is open, assess airflow. If the airway is clear, airflow is quiet and there is free movement of air. Use suction, if necessary. If you suspect severe airway obstruction from a foreign body, perform abdominal thrusts or chest compressions (depending on whether the patient is responsive or unresponsive) in adults and children, and back-blows and chest-thrusts in infants (chest compressions for the unresponsive infant). If these maneuvers are not effective, attempt to visualize the airway under direct laryngoscopy and remove the foreign body with Magill forceps. Airway edema has several causes and the treatment depends on the cause. Assess the need for advanced airway management and medications. Consider the need for intubation or supraglottic airways and cricothyroidotomy.

e. **Assess and manage breathing**   **p. 27**

Determine whether a patient has adequate breathing. Signs of inadequate breathing include altered mental status, confusion, apprehension, or agitation; shortness of breath; supraclavicular, suprasternal, or intercostal retractions; asymmetric chest wall movement; accessory muscle use; cyanosis; audible sounds (stridor, wheezing, coughing, rhonchi); abnormal respiratory rate or depth; and nasal flaring. If necessary, assist the patient's breathing with a bag-mask device or use continuous positive airway pressure (CPAP). Administer oxygen, if necessary, to maintain a SpO_2 of 95 percent or above. Cover open chest wounds with an occlusive dressing sealed on three sides, and manage tension pneumothorax with needle chest decompression.

f. **Assess and manage circulation**   **pp. 27–28**

Assess the pulse and skin to determine perfusion status and control external hemorrhage. The presence of a radial pulse suggests a systolic blood pressure of at least 80 mmHg. If the radial pulse is absent, but a carotid pulse is present, it suggests a systolic blood pressure of at least 60 mmHg. If the carotid pulse is absent, begin chest compressions and apply defibrillator pads. Assess the pulse rate, strength, and quality. You may need to treat heart-rate-related perfusion problems with medication. External hemorrhage is generally controllable with direct pressure. In some cases, topical hemostatic agents may be indicated. Severe hemorrhage in an extremity that cannot be controlled with direct pressure requires the use of a tourniquet. Depending on the underlying cause of poor perfusion, some patients may require intravenous (IV) fluids or vasopressor medications to improve perfusion. Patients with internal hemorrhage require immediate transport to a facility that can provide definitive care to control the hemorrhage.

g. **Determine priorities of care and transport**   **p. 29**

Patients who have altered mental status or problems with their airway, breathing, or circulation are a high priority for transport. For trauma patients, application of the guidelines for field triage of injured patients will help determine whether patients should be transported to a trauma center.

10. **Determine when to repeat the primary assessment.**   **p. 21**

The frequency of reassessment depends on the patient's overall condition and potential for deterioration. Patients who are critical or unstable should be reassessed more frequently. Reassess patients whenever there is a change in condition or complaint.

Case Study Review

Reread the case study on page 20 in Paramedic Care: Patient Assessment. *This case study gives you the opportunity to review the elements of the primary patient assessment process.*

EMS providers Andy and Diane have responded to a woman in her 30s who jumped from a fourth-floor balcony to the marble floor below. Their general impression reveals a patient lying in a pool of blood with obviously critical injuries. The mechanism of injury requires immediate manual stabilization of the cervical spine and the use of a jaw-thrust maneuver to open the airway. The patient is unresponsive and Andy immediately evaluates the airway. Gurgling noises and the presence of blood indicate the need for suctioning to clear the airway. Once the airway is clear, Andy focuses on assessing breathing. The patient's rapid, shallow breathing requires intervention. Diane inserts an oropharyngeal airway and ventilates the patient with a bag-mask device. Andy quickly determines the presence of chest injuries that could be contributing to the patient's poor ventilations. He checks for signs of tension pneumothorax, but does not find any. In addition to external bleeding, the patient has several indications of internal hemorrhage and shock. With the assistance of additional responders, Andy and Diane prepare the patient for immediate transport. They reassess the patient en route, and obtain a full set of vital signs.

In this case study, you observe how Andy and Diane stick to the priorities of the primary assessment to identify and immediately intervene in life-threatening problems with the airway, breathing, and circulation. They immediately recognized a critical patient in need of transport to a facility with surgical capabilities. After taking steps to address the airway and breathing, and determining the presence of shock, Andy and Diane appropriately delayed detailed assessment and IV therapy until they were en route to the hospital.

Content Self-Evaluation

MULTIPLE CHOICE

_____ 1. The primary assessment includes all of the following EXCEPT
   A. forming a general impression of the patient.
   B. stabilizing the cervical spine as needed.
   C. immobilizing fractures.
   D. assessing the airway.
   E. assessing the circulation.

_____ 2. The general patient impression is based on all of the following EXCEPT
   A. blood pressure.
   B. mechanism of injury.
   C. chief complaint.
   D. the environment.
   E. your instincts.

_____ 3. Which of the following is NOT a purpose served by your initial introduction to the patient?
   A. Identifying yourself
   B. Identifying your reason for being there
   C. Establishing your level of training
   D. Giving the patient an opportunity to refuse care
   E. Establishing informed consent

_____ 4. During the primary assessment, the cervical spine should be stabilized
   A. after the airway is established.
   B. just before you attempt artificial ventilation.
   C. immediately, if suggested by the MOI.
   D. after the circulation check.
   E. as the last step of the primary assessment.

_____ 5. Which of the following conditions is NOT a cause of altered mental status?
   A. Sleeping
   B. Drug overdose
   C. Head injury
   D. Poisoning
   E. Sepsis

_____ 6. A patient who moves only his arm when firmly pinched between the thumb and first finger and shows no other responses will be classified as which of the following under the AVPU system?
   A. A
   B. V
   C. P
   D. U
   E. Cannot be determined with the information at hand

_____ 7. A patient opens his eyes to your voice, but is disoriented and confused would be classified as which of the following under the AVPU system?
   A. A
   B. V
   C. P
   D. U
   E. Cannot be determined with the information at hand

_____ **8.** Stridor can be caused by all of the following EXCEPT
     A. infection.
     B. gastric distress.
     C. foreign body.
     D. severe swelling.
     E. allergic reaction.

_____ **9.** For stridor that is caused by respiratory burns, the care procedure most likely to maintain the airway is
     A. suctioning.
     B. blow-by oxygen and a quiet ride to the hospital.
     C. a surgical airway.
     D. early endotracheal intubation.
     E. vasoconstrictor medications.

_____ **10.** A patient with abnormally deep respirations is said to be
     A. hyperpneic.
     B. tachypneic.
     C. eupneic.
     D. bradypneic.
     E. hypopneic.

_____ **11.** The presence of a radial pulse suggests that the systolic blood pressure is at least:
     A. 60 mmHg.
     B. 70 mmHg.
     C. 80 mmHg.
     D. 100 mmHg.
     E. 120 mmHg.

_____ **12.** You apply a painful stimulus to a patient who did not respond to verbal stimuli. He rigidly extends both his arms and his legs. The response is known as _____ posturing.
     A. decorticate
     B. decerebrate
     C. purposeful
     D. noxious
     E. lethargic

_____ **13.** The greatest concern when caring for a patient with a decreased level of responsiveness is the inability of the patient to
     A. give informed consent.
     B. control his heart rate.
     C. swallow medications.
     D. give a chief complaint.
     E. protect his airway.

_____ **14.** The preferred method of initially opening the airway of an unresponsive patient without a significant mechanism of injury is a(n)
     A. modified jaw-thrust maneuver.
     B. triple airway maneuver.
     C. head-tilt/chin-lift maneuver.
     D. needle cricothyroidotomy.
     E. insertion of an oropharyngeal airway.

_____ **15.** For an unresponsive adult who has a pulse but who has inadequate breathing, you should provide bag-mask ventilations at a rate of _____ per minute.
     A. 6 to 8
     B. 8 to 10
     C. 10 to 12
     D. 12 to 16
     E. 16 to 20

_____ **16.** The presence of a basilar skull fracture is an absolute contraindication to the use of a nasopharyngeal airway.
     A. True
     B. False

_____ 17. Which of the following is correct with regard to the administration of oxygen in the primary assessment?
  A. Never apply oxygen in the primary assessment.
  B. Only apply oxygen in the primary assessment if the patient requires ventilatory assistance.
  C. Provide only enough oxygen to correct hypoxia.
  D. Always use a nonrebreather mask to administer 15 lpm of oxygen to patients who have an SpO_2 of less than 95 percent.
  E. Patients only require oxygen if the respiratory rate is below normal.

_____ 18. A respiratory rate of _____ per minute is outside the normal range for a preschool child.
  A. 20   D. 30
  B. 22   E. 34
  C. 26

_____ 19. You should suspect a problem with circulation if the heart rate of a school-age child is above _____ per minute.
  A. 110   D. 80
  B. 100   E. 70
  C. 90

_____ 20. The goal of the primary assessment is to find all problems a patient may have.
  A. True
  B. False

LISTING

List the steps of the primary assessment.

21. _____

22. _____

23. _____

24. _____

25. _____

26. _____

27. _____

Special Project

Assessing the Mental Status

Describe the findings associated with each of the letters in the AVPU mnemonic for assessing the mental status.

A. _____

V. _____

P. _____

U. _____

©2013 Pearson Education, Inc.
Paramedic Care: Principles & Practice, Vol. 3, 4th Ed.

Chapter

3

Therapeutic Communications

Review of Chapter Objectives

After reading this chapter, you should be able to:

1. **Define key terms introduced in this chapter.**

   Knowing and being able to apply the key terms in each chapter is critical to understanding chapter concepts. Write the list of key terms. Then write the definition of each one in your own words. Check your understanding by confirming the definitions in the text glossary. Correct any misunderstandings. Create a study aid by writing each key term on the front of an index card and the definition on the back. Use the cards to quiz yourself, or to have someone quiz you.

2. **Explain the critical role of therapeutic communication in EMS.** p. 37

   As a representative of emergency medical services (EMS), you are granted a certain amount of the public's trust at each new emergency scene. You must earn the rest by putting your patient and others at ease and by letting them know you are on their side, you respect their comments, and you want to help. Little courtesies, such as asking your patient his name and thereafter pronouncing it correctly, can help to accomplish this goal. Another way is by recognizing and responding with compassion to signs of discomfort or suffering. When trust is established, rapport follows. Your patients will form an opinion about you within the first few minutes, so you must establish a positive rapport quickly.

3. **Differentiate between effective and ineffective therapeutic communication strategies.** p. 37

   Effective therapeutic communication strategies you will use include persistently paying attention to word choices, tones of voice, facial expressions, and body language. You will learn to minimize external and internal distractions and to adjust your personal communication style to fit each new situation, especially when dealing with children, elderly people, people of different cultures, and hostile people.

   Unfortunately, partial or complete failure to communicate often occurs as a result of ineffective communication.

   There are abundant reasons for this, some seen in EMS are:

   - Prejudice, or lack of empathy, particularly by the paramedic toward the patient or situation
   - Lack of privacy, which inhibits a patient's responses to questions
   - External distractions, such as traffic, crowds, loud music, EMS radios, or TVs
   - Internal distractions, or thinking about things other than the situation at hand

4. **Use the basic model of communication (sender, message, receiver, feedback) to analyze therapeutic communication.** p. 37

Communication consists of a sender, a message, a receiver, and feedback. First, the sender has to encode or create, a message; that is, he must write, speak, or otherwise place symbols common to both parties in an understandable format. This may mean translating the message into another language, using words a child can understand, or writing the words on paper. The receiver must then decode, or interpret, the message, ideally with the same meaning the sender intended to convey. Finally, the receiver gives the sender feedback—a response to the message. If, by way of this response, the sender believes the message was received accurately, both parties can congratulate themselves on communicating successfully.

5. **Take actions that decrease barriers to effective therapeutic communication.** p. 43

Aside from failure to use effective techniques of therapeutic communication, barriers to communication include cultural differences, language differences, deafness, speech impediments, and even blindness. When you encounter such obstacles, try to enlist someone who can communicate with your patient and act as an interpreter. An alternative is to adopt a conservative approach toward assessment, field diagnosis, and treatment, concentrating on just the crucial items.

6. **Demonstrate interactions that build trust and rapport with others.** pp. 37–38

Building trust and rapport begins with presenting yourself as a caring, compassionate, competent, and confident health care professional. The patient will initially judge these characteristics based on your appearance, including your expression, posture, dress, and grooming. Your voice and body language must also reflect those characteristics.

Take specific steps that build trust and rapport by:

- Positioning yourself at the patient's eye-level
- Attending to the patient's needs, such as pain relief, comfort, and privacy
- Introducing yourself
- Using your patient's name and addressing him properly
- Modulating your voice and using a professional but compassionate tone
- Explaining what you are doing and why
- Keeping a kind, calm facial expression

7. **Demonstrate effective use of nonverbal communication in interactions with others.** pp. 38–40

Types of nonverbal communication include your body language, eye contact, and a compassionate touch. Your patients will pick up on your nonverbal cues through your interaction with them, so it is important to be aware of them. Body language consists of gestures, mannerisms, and postures. Your position within the environment and in relation to your patient is part of that language. Examples include distance, relative level, and stance. When interviewing your patient, make sure you look at him frequently. By doing so you can send a message to your patient such as "I care about you," or that you need the patient to "settle down now." Also be aware of circumstances that call for a compassionate touch, such as holding your patient's hand or giving him a hug. Nothing builds trust and rapport, or calms patients, faster than the power of touch.

8. **Respond effectively to patients' nonverbal behaviors.** pp. 39–42

Be aware of your patient's body language. For example, if your patient exhibits a closed stance you may be making him feel vulnerable or defensive, and you may need to change your approach. Behaviors such as fixing one's hair or other mannerisms may also tell you that your patient is uncomfortable or needs reassurance.

9. **Given a variety of scenarios, select effective questioning and active listening techniques for patient interviews.** pp. 40–42

In patient interviews you need to identify the patient's chief complaint, learn the circumstances that caused the emergency, and determine the patient's condition. Most of your answers will be accomplished by asking questions, observing the patient, listening effectively, and using appropriate language. You can begin by asking open-ended questions, and follow up, if needed, by asking direct questions to gain specific information. Avoid leading questions that end up distracting you and your patient from the emergency. Ask one question at a time and give the patient time to answer. Listen to and consider the patient's response before asking the next question. Use language the patient can understand, which often means leaving out technical medical terms that most will not be familiar with. If possible, do not allow interruptions. Learn and use active listening techniques, such as allowing silence, reflection, facilitation, empathy, clarification, confrontation, interpretation, asking about feelings, explanation, and summarization.

10. **Avoid common mistakes that can occur during patient interviews.** p. 42

Traps of interviewing, or common errors made when listening and providing feedback to patients, include the following: providing false assurances, giving advice, abusing authority, using avoidance language, distancing, using professional jargon, talking too much, interrupting, and using "why" questions. By being familiar with these errors, you can be more attentive to preventing them while on a call. You should also practice various scenarios with classmates or other professionals to be better prepared.

11. **Adapt communication strategies to communicate effectively with the following types of patients:**

   a. **Patients of all ages** pp. 44–45
   You should have an understanding of the developmental stages so you can use appropriate language and explanations for all age groups. Your patients will often be anxious, so take special care to explain everything you are doing. Be aware of prejudices you may have regarding the patient, and be patient with elderly patients, who may need additional time to process information and respond.

   b. **Patients of various cultures** p. 46
   As a nation, the United States has a diverse population in terms of culture. It is sometimes difficult to anticipate that people from backgrounds unlike yours will interpret your language and mannerisms quite differently than you intend them. Be aware of the cultural diversity in your community and learn the customs and concerns of those cultures in order to provide the best care possible.

   c. **Patients with sensory impairments** p. 45
   Blind patients, including sighted patients whose injuries may require covering the eyes, present special problems. You must identify yourself immediately, because they cannot see your uniform. Always announce yourself and explain who you are and why you are there. Remember that nonverbal communications, such as hand gestures, facial expressions, and body language, are useless in these cases. Your voice and touch are the only communication tools. The challenge of communicating with a person with a hearing impairment is much like that of overcoming a language barrier. Ask hearing-impaired and deaf patients their preferred method of communication: lip reading, signing, or writing.

   d. **Angry, hostile, uncooperative, silent, or overly talkative patients** pp. 45–47
   Anger is a natural part of the grieving process, and patients may be merely venting their frustration. Try to accept their feelings without getting defensive or angry in return.

   Set limits and establish boundaries with an uncooperative patient. If the patient is sexually aggressive, clarify your professional role for the patient. Be sure to document unusual situations. If a patient is blatantly hostile, or there is any hint that your safety is jeopardized, be sure to stay far enough away from the patient. Monitor the patient closely. To prevent a hostile situation from getting worse, be sure to have an appropriate show of force. Remember, your personal safety is paramount. Do not hesitate to involve law enforcement, if necessary.

   Some patients are excessively talkative under stress, whereas some just need someone to talk to. The problem does not have a perfect solution. You may get a less comprehensive history. Focus on important aspects and use closed-ended questions, if necessary, to keep the patient focused. Avoid becoming impatient.

e. **Patients who are anxious, crying, or depressed** pp. 47–48

Acknowledge the patient's emotions with a statement such as, "I see you are concerned about this. Do you want to talk about it?" Accept that patients are often under tremendous stress, and crying can be a response to that stress. Be supportive and quietly accepting. Depressed patients may have difficulty speaking. If you suspect depression or if the patient tells you he is depressed, ask directly about thoughts of suicide.

f. **Patients who offer multiple complaints of symptoms** p. 47

Some patients with multiple symptoms require further evaluation to determine if the source of the complaints is psychosocial or physiological. In many cases, you can narrow down the patient's chief complaint by asking what particular problem caused the patient to call for help on this occasion.

g. **Intoxicated patients** p. 48

An intoxicated patient's mood can change suddenly. Be alert to the potential for violence and protect your own safety. Be friendly and nonjudgmental. Focus on what the patient says, and not how he says it.

h. **Patients with confusing behaviors or histories** p. 48

In these cases, do not spend too much time trying to get a detailed history, because you will only become more frustrated. Focus on the mental status exam, with special emphasis on level of response, orientation, and memory.

i. **Patients with limited intelligence** p. 48

You can usually obtain an adequate history from a patient with limited intelligence. Do not assume that he will not be able to provide accurate information, but do not overlook obvious omissions because your patient appears to be giving you a good story. Evaluate your patient's education and mental abilities. If you suspect severe mental retardation, obtain the patient's history from family members.

12. **Approach sensitive topics effectively in patient interviews.** p. 46

Paramedic students normally have difficulty questioning their patients about embarrassing, sensitive, or very personal topics such as sexual activities, death and dying, physical deformities, bodily functions, and domestic violence. Even though you may feel uneasy discussing these matters, they can help you learn important information about your patient's illness. To become more comfortable dealing with these subjects, watch experienced clinicians discuss them with their patients. Familiarize yourself with and practice some opening questions on sensitive topics that both put your patient at ease and encourage him to talk about it.

13. **Provide appropriate reassurance when interacting with patients.** p. 48

Appropriate reassurance is a cornerstone of patient care. You must be careful, however, not to be overly reassuring or to prematurely reassure your anxious patient. It is natural to say, "Relax, everything is going to be all right," but your patient may have anxiety about something of which you are not aware. For instance, if your chest pain patient is anxious, you might naturally assume he is apprehensive about dying. In reality, he may be anxious about something entirely different. Now he may decide you are not interested in what is really bothering him and block further communication. Listen carefully to your patient before offering reassurance.

14. **Incorporate information from family and friends into the history when appropriate.** p. 49

Family and friends can be useful sources of information who can give you information that the patient is unable to give. However, make patient confidentiality a priority when speaking with a family member, friend, or bystander.

15. **Interact effectively with the patient's family and friends.** p. 36

Families of patients are a special group. They are concerned and worried about their loved one, and need care, too. They expect us to take good care of their loved one. They want to be kept informed. Tell them the truth and never give them false promises. Sometimes they need advice and direction. Remember that they are in crisis and may not be processing information normally. A little kindness goes a long way.

16. Communicate effectively with other health care providers to transfer care of the patient to them.

p. 49

Remember to always interact with other emergency colleagues with respect and dignity, but make sure you get the information you need, and that the person you are transferring care of the patient to listens to what you have to say.

Case Study Review

Reread the case study on pages 35–36 in Paramedic Care: Patient Assessment. *This case study draws attention to the importance of professionalism in communication.*

The paramedic student in the case study had the opportunity to observe how two different teams of EMS personnel interacted with patients and families. In the first case, the EMS providers' callous comments and actions betrayed the trust and confidence of the family and gave the paramedic student a negative impression of EMS. In the second situation, the EMS providers' actions inspired the trust and confidence of the patient and family, and left a positive impression on the student.

Content Self-Evaluation

MULTIPLE CHOICE

_____ **1.** Which of the following is an example of an open-ended question?
   A. Does your chest pain increase with breathing?
   B. Do you take diuretics?
   C. What does your pain feel like?
   D. Does the pain radiate to your shoulder?
   E. Have you had pain like this before?

_____ **2.** Which of the following questions is an example of a closed-ended question?
   A. What does your pain feel like?
   B. What were you doing when the pain started?
   C. Is your pain stabbing in nature?
   D. Why did you call us today?
   E. Where do you hurt?

_____ **3.** Always use a patient's first name during the interview to establish a closer, more trusting relationship.
   A. True
   B. False

_____ **4.** It is best to form a prearranged list of specific questions to ensure you cover all bases while interviewing your patient.
   A. True
   B. False

_____ **5.** The process of presenting the patient with an observation that he is hiding or masking the truth is called
   A. empathy.   D. clarification.
   B. confrontation.   E. facilitation.
   C. reflection.

6. Which of the following would you attempt with a patient who suddenly goes silent?
   A. Stay calm and observe for nonverbal clues.
   B. Arrange for air medical transport.
   C. Terminate the interview immediately.
   D. Attempt to walk the patient back and forth a few times.
   E. Rapidly provide oral glucose.

7. Crying is a form of venting emotional stress; be patient and provide a patient who is crying with supportive remarks.
   A. True
   B. False

8. When responding to a call that involves a small child, it is important to
   A. only speak to the parent.
   B. tell the children what you are doing and why.
   C. yell at the child if he begins to cry.
   D. involve the child in decision making whenever possible.
   E. B and D

MATCHING

Write the letter of the interview technique in the space provided next to the appropriate description.

A. empathy

B. confrontation

C. reflection

D. facilitation

E. clarification

_____ 9. Repeating the patient's words

_____ 10. Using "go on" or "I'm listening"

_____ 11. Asking questions about the patient's statements

_____ 12. Showing you understand or feel for the patient

_____ 13. Challenging a patient's statement

4

History Taking

Review of Chapter Objectives

After reading this chapter, you should be able to:

1. **Define key terms introduced in this chapter.**

   Knowing and being able to apply the key terms in each chapter is critical to understanding chapter concepts. Write the list of key terms. Then write the definition of each one in your own words. Check your understanding by confirming the definitions in the text glossary. Correct any misunderstandings. Create a study aid by writing each key term on the front of an index card and the definition on the back. Use the cards to quiz yourself, or to have someone quiz you.

2. **Apply strategies of therapeutic communication to the history-taking process.**   **p. 53**

   The ability to elicit a good history is the foundation for providing good care to patients you have never met before. To conduct a good interview, you must present yourself as a caring professional and gain your patient's trust in just a very short time. Then, you must ask the right questions, listen intently to your patient's answers, and respond accordingly.

3. **Explain the importance of both structure and flexibility in the approach to history taking.**   **p. 53**

   The medical history is a well-structured but flexible tool. In reality, your patient's answers will alter the sequence of your questioning, and not all components of a comprehensive history lend themselves well to prehospital medicine. Clinical experience is required to learn what components of the history are relevant to particular situations. Considerations in adapting the history include whether the patient is critical or non-critical, and whether the problem is medical or trauma. The chief complaint also determines the focus of the history-taking process in the prehospital setting. The situation will dictate the scope and depth of the history.

4. **Use the process of critical thinking to obtain the following components of a patient history and tailor the history-taking process based on the information obtained:**

   a. **Preliminary data**   **p. 54**

   Preliminary data include the date and time of the physical exam and history, and the patient's age, sex, race, birthplace, and occupation. Record whether the patient or someone else provided the information.

   b. **Chief complaint**   **p. 54**

   The chief complaint is the pain, discomfort, or dysfunction that caused a patient to seek help. The chief complaint is not the same as the dispatch information, or what you believe to be wrong with the patient. The chief complaint is best obtained by asking an open-ended question about the reason for the call for help. When a patient offers a chief complaint, record it in his own words.

c. Present problem
pp. 54–56

The present problem is the situation surrounding the chief complaint and call for help, and is explored by determining more information about the chief complaint and additional complaints. The mnemonic OPQRST-ASPN is useful in determining information about the present problem. By knowing the present problem you have a better idea of what happened prior to your arrival. This helps you to then begin narrowing down your working field diagnosis.

d. Past medical history
pp. 56–57

A patient's past medical history can provide significant insights into his chief complaint and help with your field diagnosis. Parts of the past medical history that can be helpful include: the general state of health, childhood diseases, adult diseases, current medications, allergies, psychiatric illnesses, accidents or injuries, and surgeries or hospitalizations. Your patient's condition, the current situation, and time constraints limit the amount of information you can attain. Use the chief complaint and present problem as a guide to make sure you obtain the most relevant information.

e. Family and social history
pp. 57–58

Aspects of a patient's family history and social history can be important in some situations, as they can indicate underlying factors that may play a role in the patient's condition. Given the circumstances, factors of the family history that you should consider are a history of heart disease, diabetes, high cholesterol, high blood pressure, stroke, kidney disease, tuberculosis, cancer, arthritis, anemia, allergies, asthma, headaches, epilepsy, mental illness, alcoholism, drug addiction, and any symptoms similar to those of the patient. This aspect of the history also includes information about the home and living situation, daily life, tobacco use, and use of alcohol and drugs. Other components to consider are the patient's diet, whether he has had health screening tests, immunization status, sleep habits, exercise, environment, use of safety measures, important experiences, religious beliefs, and the patient's outlook.

f. Review of body systems
pp. 59–60

A review of body systems is designed to identify problems your patient has not yet mentioned. General aspects include the patient's weight and any recent changes in weight, and the presence of weakness, fatigue, fever, chills, or night sweats. Ask about problems with the skin, hair, and nails; head, eyes, ears, nose, and throat; chest and lungs, heart and blood vessels; lymph nodes; gastrointestinal system; genitourinary system and male and female genitalia; musculoskeletal, neurologic, hematologic, and endocrine systems; and any psychiatric symptoms. Again, your patient's chief complaint and current status dictate how much of this information needs to be collected and what areas to pay more attention to.

5. **Apply mnemonics critically as a tool for assisting in obtaining a thorough, relevant history.**
pp. 54–56

Mnemonics abound in medicine. In this chapter you were introduced to the mnemonic OPQRST-ASPN as a way of remembering the questions used to explore the patient's chief complaint. However, mnemonics do not replace the need to carefully formulate the questions designed to get the desired information; nor do they serve as a script for asking questions. In fact, if you have listened carefully to your patient, he may already have provided you with some of the information contained in the mnemonic.

6. **Use sound clinical reasoning to develop a list of differential diagnoses based on the scene size-up, primary assessment, and medical history, and plan patient interventions.**
pp. 60–61

You must be able to gather and sort through a tremendous amount of information in a short time and make sense of it. Analyzing this data requires the total of your education, training, and clinical experience. You will sort the features of the patient's presentation into categories that contain similar features in a process called differential diagnosis. You will further narrow down the patient's problem to the pattern it fits best and arrive at a field impression for which you will develop a treatment plan. Core components of the clinical reasoning process include your base of knowledge and skills, the ability to gather data, the process of forming differential diagnoses, the ability to sort through and manage ambiguous information, recognizing patterns, and being able to defend your decisions.

©2013 Pearson Education, Inc.
Paramedic Care: Principles & Practice, Vol. 3, 4th Ed.

Case Study Review

Reread the case study on page 52 in Paramedic Care: Patient Assessment. *This case study draws attention to the value of the information gathered during the patient history and the process by which it is obtained.*

The investigation of the chief complaint, associated symptoms, and past medical history is extremely important both in determining what is wrong with your patient and in guiding your provision of care. The circumstances of the emergency and the patient's presentation may confound you unless you employ a relatively standard, systematic approach to patient questioning. Questioning must remain flexible enough to adapt to different circumstances. In a trauma emergency, you examine the mechanism of injury to determine what happened, whereas with a medical patient you must investigate the current and past medical history in depth.

Paramedic supervisor Dan Colbert is presented with an "elderly man with abdominal pain."

He begins his investigation of the history by introducing himself, identifying his role at the scene, and expressing his desire to help Mr. O'Mara. He also asks for and uses Mr. O'Mara's name to place the conversation on a more comfortable and personal level.

Dan first determines the patient's chief complaint, the problem that led him to call for the ambulance. (This may differ from the primary problem in some cases.) In this case, the chief complaint is "My stomach hurts." Dan then quickly investigates the complaint by asking questions. The questions he asks are extensive and systematically examine the patient's symptoms. Note that these questions follow the acronym OPQRST-ASPN. Dan questions about onset *(What were you doing when it started? Did it come on suddenly?),* provocation/palliation *(Does anything make it better or worse?),* quality *(Can you describe how it feels?),* radiation *(Can you point to the area that hurts? Does the pain travel anywhere else?),* severity *(How bad is it? On a scale of one to ten, with ten being the worst pain you have ever felt, how would you rate this pain?),* time *(When did it start? Is it constant or does it come and go?),* and associated symptoms and pertinent negatives *(Are you nauseous and have you vomited? Have you experienced a change in your bowel habits? Do you have any difficulty breathing?).* As Dan asks these questions, he leans forward and repeats parts of the patient's answers to show his interest and involvement.

The approach that Dan uses ensures an ordered and in-depth investigation of all elements of the patient's history. At the emergency scene, there is much going on and often a sense of urgency. However, taking the few moments to inquire about the patient's presentation ensures that you have the essential information to begin forming a differential field diagnosis.

Based on what he has discovered, Dan begins to form his differential field diagnosis. Although the history of pain immediately after eating suggests gallbladder problems (cholecystitis), Dan suspects a broader list of potential problems. This keeps him from forming tunnel vision. As he investigates the past medical history, he asks questions to support or rule out these other problems.

Dan questions Mr. O'Mara about his past medical history and gains further information about pain after eating fatty foods, indigestion, and alcohol consumption. The patient's denials of bloody emesis and stools are pertinent negatives that help Dan rule out other possible diagnoses. This information also helps him confirm a final field diagnosis of gallbladder problems. With the facts that support his evaluation, Dan conveys the results of his patient questioning to Dr. Cooney at the emergency department. The laboratory findings support the field diagnosis, and Mr. O'Mara is quickly moved to surgery.

Content Self-Evaluation

MULTIPLE CHOICE

_____ 1. In the majority of medical cases, the basis of the paramedic's field diagnosis is the
   A. chief complaint.
   B. index of suspicion.
   C. mechanism of injury.
   D. patient history.
   E. vital signs.

_____ 2. A good paramedic asks the same questions of every patient, in the same order every time.
   A. True
   B. False

_____ 3. It is NOT necessary to reconfirm information with a patient if you received the initial information from a health care provider.
   A. True
   B. False

_____ 4. The list of possible causes for a patient's symptoms is the
   A. index of suspicion.
   B. mechanism of injury.
   C. differential field diagnosis.
   D. CAGE questionnaire.
   E. nature of the illness.

_____ 5. It is appropriate, if not necessary, to take notes while interviewing the patient because it is nearly impossible to remember everything important the patient tells you.
   A. True
   B. False

_____ 6. In the mnemonic OPQRST-ASPN, which aspect describes the question, "Where is your discomfort? Does it move?"
   A. Onset
   B. Quality
   C. Region/Radiation
   D. Time
   E. Severity

_____ 7. The chief complaint and primary problem are interchangeable terms.
   A. True
   B. False

_____ 8. The mnemonic OPQRST-ASPN is used to obtain the patient's past medical history.
   A. True
   B. False

_____ 9. Which of the following would be recorded as a palliating factor with regard to a patient's chief complaint?
   A. Nausea increases in response to movement.
   B. The pain is the same as it was when the patient had a gallbladder attack.
   C. Difficulty breathing is decreased when the patient sits or stands up.
   D. Abdominal discomfort is worse after the patient eats or drinks.
   E. Bloody stools have been going on for three days.

_____ 10. The reason (pain, discomfort, or dysfunction) that the patient or another person summons emergency medical services is termed the
   A. primary problem.
   B. chief complaint.
   C. nature of the illness.
   D. mechanism of injury.
   E. none of the above.

_____ 11. The underlying cause of the patient's pain, discomfort, or dysfunction is called the
   A. primary problem.
   B. chief complaint.
   C. nature of the illness.
   D. mechanism of injury.
   E. none of the above.

_____ 12. Any activity that alleviates a patient's symptoms would fit under which element of the OPQRST-ASPN mnemonic for the history of the current illness?
   A. O
   B. The first P
   C. Q
   D. R
   E. The second P

_____ **13.** Which of the following is an important part of the past medical history?
- **A.** Radiation of the pain
- **B.** Last oral intake
- **C.** Surgeries or hospitalizations
- **D.** Quality of the pain
- **E.** All of the above

_____ **14.** A recently prescribed medication may account for medical problems because of which of the following?
- **A.** Overmedication
- **B.** Undermedication
- **C.** Allergic reaction
- **D.** Untoward reaction
- **E.** All of the above

_____ **15.** Allergies should be expected for all of the following EXCEPT
- **A.** the "caine" family.
- **B.** tetanus toxoid.
- **C.** glucose.
- **D.** narcotics.
- **E.** both A and B.

_____ **16.** A patient who has smoked 21 packs of cigarettes a week for 10 years has a pack history of
- **A.** 21 pack/years.
- **B.** 70 pack/years.
- **C.** 7 pack/years.
- **D.** 30 pack/years.
- **E.** 10 pack/years.

_____ **17.** Which of the following is a system examined during the review of systems?
- **A.** Skin
- **B.** Lymphatic system
- **C.** Musculoskeletal system
- **D.** Hematologic system
- **E.** All of the above are examined

_____ **18.** While reviewing the patient history form provided to you when you picked up your patient at a physician's office, you note the documentation G2P1A0L1. From this you know that the patient
- **A.** is currently pregnant and has one living child.
- **B.** is currently pregnant and lost one child.
- **C.** had one past pregnancy and one miscarriage.
- **D.** had one normal pregnancy and one complicated pregnancy.
- **E.** has had one pregnancy that resulted in twins.

_____ **19.** Which of the following is NOT necessary for effective clinical reasoning?
- **A.** The ability to gather data
- **B.** The ability to sort relevant from irrelevant data
- **C.** A fund of knowledge about pathophysiology and expected normal findings
- **D.** The ability to compare a patient's presentation with that of other patients you have seen
- **E.** The ability to come to a definitive diagnosis for all patients

MATCHING

Write the letter of the body system in the space provided next to the question designed to review that system.

A. endocrine

B. neurologic

C. musculoskeletal

D. hematologic

E. chest and lungs

_____ **20.** Have you ever had pneumonia?

_____ **21.** Do you have any pain in your joints?

_____ **22.** Have you been unusually fatigued?

_____ **23.** Do you have any problems with memory?

_____ **24.** Have you been excessively thirsty recently?

Classify each question or statement under the OPQRST category that best applies by writing the letter of the category in the space provided.

O. onset

P. provocation/palliation

Q. quality

R. region/radiation

S. severity

T. time

_____ **25.** How does this compare to the worst pain you have ever felt?

_____ **26.** Does rest lessen your pain?

_____ **27.** Point to where you feel pain.

_____ **28.** Does this pain feel crushing in nature?

_____ **29.** Does deep breathing increase the pain?

_____ **30.** Did this pain begin suddenly or gradually?

_____ **31.** Where does this pain travel to?

_____ **32.** When did the first symptoms begin?

_____ **33.** Describe how the pain feels.

_____ **34.** Were you walking or running when this pain first began?

SHORT ANSWER

35. Compare and contrast the differential field diagnosis and the final field diagnosis.

_____

_____

_____

_____

Special Project

History of the Present Illness

Read the following narrative description of a patient history, and then organize the information into the OPQRST-ASPN format.

At just about noon, your unit, Rescue 31, responds to a "man down" call at a local park. You arrive to find an approximately 20-year-old male on the ground surrounded by onlookers. The man is sitting up and talking with a police officer. You introduce yourself and begin to form a general impression of the patient. He is articulate and appears to be conscious, alert, and fully oriented. The patient states that he was jogging when he suddenly had a sharp chest pain, became dizzy, and collapsed. He now complains of mild difficulty breathing and increased pain with deep breathing.

The patient states that the pain is very severe and ranks about 8 on a 1-to-10 scale, with 10 being the worst pain he has ever experienced. He describes the pain as stabbing and indicates its location, which is just to the left of the sternum at about the 3rd intercostal space.

©2013 Pearson Education, Inc.
Paramedic Care: Principles & Practice, Vol. 3, 4th Ed.

He denies pain anywhere else. The pain began suddenly, without warning, and he has never experienced anything like it. He denies taking a deep breath or coughing before the pain began. He says he has not had previous breathing or chest problems and says he does not have any history of chronic obstructive pulmonary disease (COPD), asthma, or heart problems. He is not currently taking any medications, nor is he being treated for any medical problem.

O. _____

_____

P. _____

_____

Q. _____

_____

R. _____

_____

S. _____

_____

T. _____

_____

AS. _____

_____

PN. _____

_____

Secondary Assessment

Review of Chapter Objectives

After reading this chapter, you should be able to:

1. Define key terms introduced in this chapter.

Knowing and being able to apply the key terms in each chapter is critical to understanding chapter concepts. Write the list of key terms. Then write the definition of each one in your own words. Check your understanding by confirming the definitions in the text glossary. Correct any misunderstandings. Create a study aid by writing each key term on the front of an index card and the definition on the back. Use the cards to quiz yourself, or to have someone quiz you.

2. Describe the general approach to physical examination. pp. 66–67

You should develop a personal order in which you assess patients, as this makes sure you do not leave out any part of the exam. Make sure that you are systematic and efficient as you move through the exam. Use your active listening techniques, and provide reassurance and compassion as needed. Your patients will often be apprehensive, so try to take steps to alleviate this by being confident and skillful in your exam.

3. Apply the techniques of inspection, palpation, percussion, and
auscultation to the physical examination process. pp. 67–70

Inspection is the process of informed observation, viewing the patient for anatomical shape, coloration, and movement. It is the least invasive examination tool yet may provide the most patient information.

Palpation is the use of touch to gather information regarding size, shape, position, temperature, moisture, texture, movement, and response to pressure. The fingertips are most sensitive, the palm best evaluates vibration, and the back of the hand is most sensitive to temperature.

Percussion is the production of a vibration in tissue to elicit sounds. These sounds—dull, resonant, hyperresonant, tympanic, and flat—identify the nature of the tissue underneath. The vibration is generated by striking the first knuckle of a finger placed against the area to be percussed with the fingertip of the other hand.

Auscultation is listening for sounds within the body, most frequently with a stethoscope. The intensity, pitch, duration, quality, and timing of sounds in the patient's lungs, heart, blood vessels, and intestines are compared against normal sounds.

4. **Interpret the findings obtained through inspection, palpation, percussion, and auscultation.** pp. 67–70

Inspection allows you to determine whether or not a patient is conscious or seems unresponsive, and allows you to detect the patient's position, obvious injuries, and many other signs of illness and injury.

During palpation you will be checking for growths, swelling, tenderness, spasms, rigidity, pain, and crepitus. Observe how your patient responds to you, as this can indicate tender areas, even in patients who are unresponsive.

Percussion provides three basic sounds: dull, resonant, and hyperresonant. Dull reflects a density and is a medium-pitched thud. It is usually caused by a dense organ (such as the liver) or fluid (such as blood) underneath. Resonant sounds are generally associated with a less dense tissue, such as the lungs, and are lower-pitched and longer-lasting sounds. Hyperresonant sounds reflect air, or air under pressure, and are the lowest-pitched sounds and the ones that diminish in volume most slowly.

Auscultation allows you to differentiate between normal and abnormal breath sounds and bowel sounds. During auscultation of the chest you may hear normal breathing, or you may hear crackles, wheezes, or rhonchi.

5. **Adapt your use of a stethoscope to the information you are seeking to obtain.** pp. 69–70

The diaphragm of the stethoscope is held firmly against the skin, while the bell is placed lightly on the skin. With light pressure, the bell picks up low-pitched sounds, such as lung sounds. The diaphragm, or the bell, if pressure is applied, screens out low-pitched sounds and allows you to hear high-pitched sounds, such as blood pressure sounds and heart sounds.

When examining the chest, have your patient breathe more deeply and slowly than normal with an open mouth. Using the stethoscope's disk, auscultate each side of the chest from the apex to the base every 5 cm, listening at each location for one full breath.

Using the diaphragm of the stethoscope, you can listen for heart sounds at the 2nd through 5th intercostal spaces at both sternal borders and at the point of maximum impulse (PMI). Repeat the process using the bell of the stethoscope to discern lower-pitched sounds.

To examine the abdomen, use the stethoscope's disk, and auscultate each abdominal quadrant for at least 30 seconds to 1 minute.

6. **Given a variety of scenarios, perform a general survey to include assessing the patient's mental status, general appearance, and vitals signs.** pp. 70–82

The general survey is the first part of the comprehensive exam. It is made up of your evaluation of the patient's appearance—including level of consciousness, expression, state of health, general characteristics (for example, weight, height), posturing, dress, grooming, and so on—the vital signs, and additional assessments, such as pulse oximetry, cardiac monitoring, and blood glucose determination. The survey helps you form a general impression of your patient's health.

The evaluation of mental status begins with your interview. The evaluation permits you to determine your patient's level of responsiveness, general appearance, behavior, and speech. You specifically look at his appearance and behavior, speech and language skills, mood, thought and perception, insight and judgment, and memory and attention.

When taking your patient's vital signs you are documenting a baseline measurement that can be compared to as you continue your assessment and reassessment. The results are primary indicators of your patient's health and must be done early on. You need to measure the respiratory, circulatory, and perfusion status. Especially in emergency situations, you need to repeat the vital signs often to look for trends. Trends can then indicate potential problems and allow you to better treat the patient. You will assess your patient's respiratory rate by counting the number of times he breathes in 1 minute. It is important to also note any effort the patient is taking to breathe, and the quality of the breaths. Another vital sign you need to measure is the pulse, and its rate, rhythm, and quality. Blood pressure, body temperature, capillary refill, and oral mucosa color are also important vital signs that must be measured.

©2013 Pearson Education, Inc.
Paramedic Care: Principles & Practice, Vol. 3, 4th Ed.

7. Interpret the meaning of findings obtained in the general survey.   **pp. 70–82**

The general survey can give a wealth of information, such as clues to the patient's mental state and possible behavioral disorders. For example, is a patient very still with a lack of facial expression, indicating that you should explore the possibility of depression? Or is the patient tense, restless, and fidgeting, indicating possible anxiety? The patient's dress, grooming, and hygiene can also tell you about the patient's mental state. The patient's general appearance may be that of a generally healthy person, or may tell you that the patient has chronic illness. Vital signs have defined normal parameters, and any deviation from them can give you information about the patient's condition.

8. Demonstrate examination of the anatomic regions of the body.

Discussed in combination with objective 9, below.

9. Interpret examination findings of the following structures and systems:

a. **Skin, hair, and nails**   **pp. 82–88**

Observe the skin carefully for color, especially in the nail beds, lips, conjunctiva, and mucous membranes of the mouth. Pink skin reflects good oxygenation, whereas pale skin reflects poor blood flow from hypovolemia, hypothermia, compensatory shock, or anemia. A bluish skin, referred to as cyanosis, suggests the blood is low in oxygen. A yellow sclera or general discoloration, termed jaundice, is due to liver failure. Other skin observations may include petechiae, which are small, round, flat, purplish spots caused by capillary bleeding from a variety of etiologies, and ecchymosis, a larger, black-and-blue discoloration that is often the result of trauma or bleeding disorders. Moisture, temperature, texture, mobility, and turgor are also evaluated. Skin lesions are disruptions in normal tissue that may take on almost any shape, color, or arrangement.

Inspect and palpate the hair to determine color, quality, distribution, quantity, and texture and inspect and palpate the scalp for scaling, lesions, redness, lumps, or tenderness. Generalized hair loss may reflect chemotherapy; failure to develop normal hair patterns may be caused by a pituitary or hormonal problem; and unusual facial hair in women suggests a hormonal imbalance. Mild scalp flaking suggests dandruff, heavy scaling suggests psoriasis, and greasy scaling suggests seborrheic dermatitis. Lice eggs (nits) may be found firmly attached to the hair shafts. Normal hair texture is smooth and soft in Caucasians; in people of African descent, the texture is coarser. Dry, brittle, or fragile hair is abnormal.

Inspect the fingernails and toenails for color. Note any discolorations, lesions, ridging, grooves, depressions, or pitting. Depressions suggest systemic disease. Compress the nail and bed to determine its adherence and look for nail hygiene. Any boggyness suggests cardiorespiratory disease.

b. **Head, ears, eyes, nose, and mouth**   **pp. 88–105**

Observe and palpate the skull and facial region for symmetry, smoothness, wounds, bleeding, size, and general contour. Examine the hair and scalp as described previously. Check the eyes for bilateral periorbital and mastoid ecchymosis, "raccoon eyes" and "Battle's sign," respectively. They suggest basilar skull fracture and occur an hour or so after injury. Palpate the facial region for crepitation, false motion, or instability suggesting fracture. Evaluate the temporomandibular joint for pain, tenderness, swelling, and range of motion. Have the patient open and close his mouth and jut and retract his jaw. Any loss of normal function suggests injury.

Examine for visual acuity, then evaluate for peripheral vision. Visual acuity is the ability to read detail. A wall chart with lines of progressively smaller letters is placed at 20 feet from the patient. He then reads to the smallest line in which he can recognize at least one-half of the letters. The result is recorded as the distance from the chart and the distance at which a person with normal sight could distinguish the letters, 20/20 for normal or 20/60 for someone who reads what is normally read at 60 feet.

While the patient faces you, have him look at your nose while you extend your arms, bend your elbows, and wiggle your fingers. If he notices the fingers moving in all four directions (up, down, left, and right) for each eye, his peripheral vision is grossly normal. Inspect the eyes for symmetry, shape, inflammation, swelling, misalignment (disconjugate gaze), lesions, and contour. Examine the eyelids, open and closed, for swelling, discoloration, droop (ptosis), styes, and lash positioning. Observe the tearing or dryness of the eyes. Gently retract the lower eyelid while asking the patient to look through a range of motion. Examine the sclera for signs of irritation, cloudiness, yellow discoloration (jaundice), any nodules, swelling, discharge, or hemorrhage into the scleral tissue. With an oblique light source, inspect the cornea for opacities. Inspect the size, shape, symmetry, and reactivity of the pupils. Note the pupils' direct and consensual response to increased light intensity. A sluggish pupil suggests pressure on CN-III; bilateral sluggishness suggests global hypoxia or depressant drug action. Constricted pupils suggest opiate overdose; dilated and fixed pupils reflect brain anoxia. Ask the patient to focus on your finger close at hand; then move the hand to his nose, then away. The eyes should converge, and the pupils should constrict slightly. Then have him follow your finger as you move it through an "H" pattern. The eyes should move smoothly together. Nystagmus is a jerky movement at the distal extremes of ocular movement. Gently touch the cornea with a strand of cotton. The patient should respond with a blink.

The ophthalmoscope is a light source and a series of lenses that permit you to examine the interior of the patient's eyes. It allows you to examine the retina, blood vessels, and optic nerve at the back of the posterior chamber of the eye. Using an ophthalmoscope, look into the eye's anterior chamber for signs of blood (hyphema), cells, or pus (hypopyon) and check the cornea for lacerations, abrasions, cataracts, papilledema (from increased intracranial pressure), vascular occlusions, and retinal hemorrhage.

Examine the ears by looking for symmetry from in front of the patient; then examine each ear separately. Examine the external portion (auricle) for shape, size, landmarks, and position on the head. Examine the surrounding area for deformities, lesions, tenderness, and erythema. Pull the helix upward and outward, press on the tragus and on the mastoid process, and note any discomfort or pain, suggesting otitis or mastoiditis. Some pain may be associated with toothache, a cold, a sore throat, or cervical spine injury. Inspect the ear canal for discharge (pus, mucus, blood, or cerebral spinal fluid [CSF]) and inflammation. Trauma can account for blood, mucus, and CSF in the ear canal. Check hearing acuity by covering one ear and whispering, then speaking into the other. Hearing loss may be accounted for by trauma, accumulation of debris (often cerumen), tympanic membrane rupture, drug use, and prolonged exposure to loud noise.

The otoscope is a light source and a magnifying lens that permit examination of a patient's ears and nose. The otoscope allows you to examine the external auditory canal and the tympanic membrane for trauma, irritation, or infection. Visualize the inner canal with the otoscope. With the largest speculum that will fit the canal, turn the patient's head away from you, pull the auricle slightly up and backward, and insert the otoscope. Inspect for wax (cerumen), discharge, redness, lesions, perforations, and foreign bodies. Then focus on the tympanic membrane. It should be a translucent pearly, white-to-pinkish gray. Color changes suggest fluid behind the eardrum, scarring, or infection. Also check for bulging, protractions, or perforations.

Visualize the patient's nose from the front and sides to determine any asymmetry, deviation, tenderness, flaring, or abnormal color. Tilt your patient's head back slightly and examine the nostrils. Insert the otoscope and check for deviation of the septum and perforations. Examine the nasal mucosa for color and the color, consistency, and quantity of drainage. Rhinitis (a runny nose) suggests seasonal allergies, a thick yellow discharge suggests infection, and blood suggests epistaxis from trauma or a septal defect. Test each side of the nose for patency by occluding the other side during a breath. There is normally some difference in patency between the sides. Palpate the frontal sinuses for swelling and tenderness.

Begin assessment of the mouth by observing the lips for color and condition. They should be pink, smooth, and symmetrical, without lesions, swelling, lumps, cracks, or scaliness. Using a bright light and tongue blade, examine the oral mucosa for color, lesions, white patches, or fissures. The mucosa should be pinkish red, smooth, and moist. The gums should be pink, with clearly defined margins around the teeth. The teeth should be well formed and straight. If the gums are swollen, bleed easily, and are separated from the teeth, suspect periodontal disease. Ask the patient to stick his tongue out and note its velvety surface. Hold the tongue with a 2-by-2-inch gauze pad and inspect all sides and the bottom. All surfaces should be pink and smooth.

Then examine the pharynx and have the patient say "aaaahhh" while you hold the tongue down with a tongue blade. Watch the movement of the uvula and the coloration and condition of the palatine tonsils and posterior pharynx. Look for any pus, swelling, ulcers, or drainage. Also notice any odors, including alcohol, feces (bowel obstruction), acetone (diabetic ketoacidosis), gastric contents, coffee-grounds-like material (gastric hemorrhage), pink-tinged sputum (pulmonary edema), or bitter almonds (cyanide poisoning).

©2013 Pearson Education, Inc.
Paramedic Care: Principles & Practice, Vol. 3, 4th Ed.

c. **Neck** pp. 103–105

Inspect your patient's neck for symmetry and visible masses. Note any deformity, deviations, tugging, scars, gland enlargement, or visible lymph nodes. Examine for any open wounds and cover them with an occlusive dressing. Examine the jugular veins for distention while the patient is seated upright and at a 45° incline. Palpate the trachea to ensure it is in line. Palpate the thyroid while the patient swallows to ensure it is small, smooth, and without nodules. Palpate each lymph node to determine size, shape, tenderness, consistency, and mobility. Tender, swollen, and mobile nodes suggest inflammation from infection; hard and fixed ones suggest malignancy.

d. **Chest and Lungs** pp. 105–111

To assess the chest, you need a stethoscope with a bell and diaphragm. Expose the entire thorax with consideration for the patient's dignity and modesty and inspect, palpate, percuss, and auscultate. Compare findings from one side of the chest to those from the other and from posterior to anterior. Look for general shape and symmetry as well as for the rate and pattern of breathing. Observe for retractions and the use of accessory muscles (suggestive of airway obstruction or restriction) and palpate for deformities, tenderness, crepitus (suggestive of rib fracture), and abnormal chest excursion (suggestive of flail chest or spinal injury). Feel for vibrations associated with air movement and speech. Percuss the chest for dullness (hemothorax, pleural effusion, or pneumonia), resonance, and hyperresonance (pneumothorax or tension pneumothorax). Finally, auscultate the lung lobes for normal breath sounds, crackles (pulmonary edema), wheezes (asthma), rhonchi, stridor (airway obstruction), and pleural friction rubs.

Chest excursion

Place your hands at the 10th intercostal space with the fingers spread and feel for chest excursion as the patient breathes deeply. Your hand should move equally about 3 to 5 cm with each breath.

Fremitus

Place a cupped hand against the chest wall at various locations and feel for vibrations while the patient says "ninety-nine" or "one-on-one." These vibrations should be equal throughout the chest. Note any enhanced, decreased, or absent fremitus.

Diaphragm excursion

Percuss the border of the rib cage for the dullness of the diaphragm during quiet breathing. Then mark the highest and lowest movement during respiration. Repeat the process on the other side of the chest. This excursion should be about 6 cm and equal on each side.

Breath sounds pp. 88–92

Normal breath sounds are the quiet sounds (almost low-pitched sighs) of air moving. Abnormal breath sounds are termed "adventitious" and include the following. Any crackles (a light crackling, popping, nonmusical sound) suggest fluid in the smaller airways. Late inspiratory crackles suggest heart failure or interstitial lung disease, whereas early crackles suggest heart failure or chronic bronchitis. Wheezes (more musical notes) denote obstruction of the smaller airways. The closer they appear to inspiration, the more serious is the obstruction. Stridor is a high-pitched, loud inspiratory wheeze reflective of laryngeal or tracheal obstruction. Grating or squeaking sounds describe pleural friction rubs and occur as the pleural layers become inflamed, then rub together. You may also listen for sound transmission while the patient speaks. Bronchophony occurs when you hear the words "ninety-nine" abnormally clearly through the stethoscope, a suggestion that blood, fluid, or a tumor has replaced normal tissue. Assess for whispered pectoriloquy by asking the patient to whisper "ninety-nine"; unusually clear sounds indicate an abnormal condition. Egophony occurs when you can hear the sound of long "e" as "a" when vocal resonance is abnormally increased.

e. **Heart and Blood Vessels** pp. 111–119

The patient's skin color provides information about the adequacy of perfusion. Inspect the neck for the pulsation of the carotid arteries and jugular vein distension, and palpate the carotid arteries. Determine the rate, rhythm, and quality of the pulse. Assess for pulsus paradoxus, thrills, and bruits. Check the patient's blood pressure and assess the peripheral pulses. Auscultate the heart sounds to

assess the function of the cardiac valves for possible indications of heart failure. Assess the extremities for edema related to heart failure and signs of deep vein thrombosis.

Locate a soft and pulsing carotid artery in the neck, just lateral to the cricoid cartilage, to avoid pressure on the carotid sinus. Carefully press down until the pulse wave just lifts your finger off the artery. Determine the rate and carefully evaluate for regularity. Irregularity may be caused by dysrhythmia, whereas variation in strength may be due to such phenomena as pulsus paradoxus, increasing strength with exhalation and decreasing with inhalation. Also note any thrills (humming or vibration) and listen with the stethoscope for bruits (sounds of turbulent flow).

Examine the anterior neck and locate the jugular veins. Position your patient with his head elevated 30° and turned away from you. Look for pulsation just above the suprasternal notch. Identify the highest point of pulsation and measure the distance from the sternal angle. The highest point of pulsation is usually between 1 and 2 cm from the sternal angle. (Distention when the patient is elevated at higher angles may reflect tension pneumothorax or pericardial tamponade, whereas flat veins at lower angles may suggest hypovolemia.)

Heart sounds

The normal heart produces a "lub-dub" sound heard through the disk of the stethoscope with each cardiac contraction. The "lub" and "dub" may split when valves close out of sync—"la-lub-dub" reflects an S1 split; "lub-da-dub" is an S2 split. S2 splitting is normal in children and young adults, though abnormal in older adults if expiratory or persistent splitting occurs. S3 splitting produces a "lub-dub-dee" cadence, such as the word "Kentucky." It occurs commonly in children and young adults but reflects blood filling a dilated ventricle and may suggest ventricular failure in the patient over 30. The S4 heart sound is the "dee" sound of "dee-lub-dub" with a cadence similar to the word "Tennessee." It develops from vibrations as the atrium pushes blood into a ventricle that resists filling, suggestive of heart failure.

Inspection for signs of cardiovascular insufficiency

Examine the extremities for signs of insufficiency, including pallor, delayed capillary refill, temperature variation, and dependent edema. Then assess the carotid arteries for pulse strength, rate, and rhythm. Does the rate or strength vary with respirations? Do you feel thrills (feel a humming sensation)? If so, auscultate for bruits.

Jugular vein distention

Position the patient supine with the head elevated 30° and turned away from the side being assessed. Look for pulsations of the external jugular vein on either side of the trachea just before it passes behind the manubrium. Locate the highest point of pulsation and measure the distance from the sternal angle. Normal venous pressure distends the vein above the clavicle between 1 and 2 cm. Examine both jugulars for symmetrical pulsing and distention.

Point of maximum impulse (PMI)

Have the patient lie comfortably with his head elevated 30°. Inspect and palpate the chest for the apical impulse, or the PMI. It is normally at the 5th intercostal space, midclavicular line. In muscular or obese patients, you may need to percuss the point (dull vs. resonant).

Heart and blood vessels

Examine the cardiovascular function by inspecting for skin pallor or other signs suggestive of arterial insufficiency or occlusion. Then evaluate carotid and peripheral pulses for rate, rhythm, and quality as well as the jugular vein for signs of distention (JVD). A heart rate above 100 is tachycardia and may be related to excitement and stress or shock, whereas a heart rate below 60 (bradycardia) may be related to an athlete's state of conditioning or head injury. Excessive JVD suggests right heart failure or cardiac tamponade, and abnormally low distention may suggest hypovolemia. Auscultate the heart sounds either side of the sternum at the 2nd intercostal space and the left side of the sternum at the 5th intercostal space. Variations of the normal "lub-dub" suggest cardiac abnormalities, though some variant sounds may be normal in children and young adults.

©2013 Pearson Education, Inc.
Paramedic Care: Principles & Practice, Vol. 3, 4th Ed.

Peripheral vascular system

Examine the upper, then the lower, extremities and compare them, one to another, for the following: size, symmetry, swelling, venous congestion, skin and nail bed color, temperature, skin texture, and turgor. Yellow and brittle nails, swollen digit ends (clubbing), or poor nail bed color suggests chronic arterial insufficiency. Assess the distal circulation, noting the strength, rate, and regularity of the pulse and comparing pulses bilaterally. If you have difficulty palpating a pulse or cannot find one, palpate a more proximal site. Feel the spongy compliance of the vessels, note their coloration, and examine for inflammation along the vein, indicative of deep vein thrombosis. Gently feel for edema and pitting edema in each distal extremity.

f. **Abdomen**   pp. 119–120

Question your patient regarding any pain, tenderness, or unusual feeling, as well as recent bowel and bladder function. Carefully inspect the area for scars, dilated veins, stretch marks, rashes, lesions, and pigmentation changes. Discoloration around the umbilicus (Cullen's sign) or over the flanks (Grey Turner's sign) suggests intra-abdominal hemorrhage. Assess the size and shape of the abdomen, determining whether it is scaphoid (concave), flat, round, or distended, and look for any bulges or hernias. Ascites results in bulges in the flanks and across the abdomen, suggesting congestive heart or liver failure, whereas suprapubic bulges suggest a full bladder or pregnant uterus. Look also for any masses, palpations, or peristalsis. A slight vascular pulsing is normal, but excessive movement suggests an aneurysm. Auscultate and percuss as described earlier. Then depress each quadrant gently and release. Look for patient expression or muscle guarding suggestive of injury or peritonitis.

Normal bowel sounds consist of a variety of high-pitched gurgles and clicks that occur every 5 to 15 seconds. More frequent activity suggests an increase in bowel motility, and especially loud and prolonged gurgling sounds (borborygmi) indicate hyperperistalsis. Decreased or absent sounds suggest a paralytic ileus or peritonitis. You may also hear swishing sounds (bruit) over the major vessels, suggesting a vascular defect, such as aneurysm or stenosis.

g. **Male and female genitalia**   pp. 124–125

Except in cases of trauma to the genitalia and in women in labor with indications of imminent delivery, the genitalia are rarely examined in the prehospital setting. Examination is limited to inspection.

h. **Anus**   pp. 125–126

Position your patient on his left side with legs flexed and buttocks near the edge of the stretcher. Be sensitive to the patient's feelings and drape or cover any areas not being observed. With a gloved hand, spread the buttocks apart and examine the area for lumps, ulcers, inflammations, rashes, or lesions. Palpate any areas carefully, noting inflammation or tenderness. If appropriate, obtain a fecal sample for testing.

i. **Musculoskeletal system**   pp. 127–145

Advancing age causes changes in the musculoskeletal system, including shortening and increased curvature of the spine, a reduction in muscle mass and strength, and a reduction in the range of motion. Observe the patient's general posture, build, and muscular development as well as the movement of the extremities, gait, and position at rest. Then inspect all regions of the body for deformities, symmetry and symmetrical movement, joint structure, and swelling, nodules, or inflammation. Deformities are often related to misaligned articulating bones, dislocations, or subluxations. Impaired movement is usually related to arthritis; nodules are related to rheumatic fever or rheumatoid arthritis; and redness is related to gout, rheumatic fever, or arthritis. Compare dissimilar joints to determine what structures might be affected. Assess range of motion by moving the limb, asking the patient to move the limb, and then asking the patient to move the limb against resistance. Note any asymmetry and inequality between active and passive motion. Also examine for crepitation (a grating vibration or sound) that may suggest arthritis, an inflamed joint, or a fracture. Avoid manipulating a deformed or painful joint. Perform a physical exam on each joint, moving it through its normal range of motion and noting any deformities, limited or resistant movement, tenderness, and swelling.

j. **Neurologic system**   pp. 146–155

Assessment of the nervous system includes determination of whether a deficit is symmetrical or unilateral and whether the deficit arises from the central or peripheral nervous system. Beyond the mental status exam conducted in the general survey, you may assess the function of the 12 pairs of cranial nerves using standard tests, and may assess the sensory and motor function of the spinal nerves. Assess for muscle tone, coordination, and positioning. Observe for tremors or tics. Testing reflexes determines the function of the reflex arcs in the spinal cord.

To evaluate mental status and speech, examine your patient's appearance and behavior, speech and language, mood, thoughts and perceptions, and memory and attention. Observe the patient's appearance and behavior, level of consciousness, posture and motor behavior, appropriateness of dress, grooming and personal hygiene, and facial expression. Note any abnormal speech pattern and observe the patient's attitude toward you and others expressed both verbally and nonverbally. Note any excessive emotion or lack of emotion. Assess the patient's thoughts and perceptions. Are they realistic and socially acceptable? Question for any visions, voices, perceived odors, or feelings about things that are not there. Examine the patient's insights and judgments to determine if he knows what is happening. Assess the patient's memory and attention and determine his orientation to time, place, and person (sometimes considered as person and own person). Then test immediate, recent, and remote memory. Any deviation from a normal and expected response is to be noted and suggests illness or a psychiatric problem.

Begin the examination of the motor system by observing the patient for symmetry, deformities, and involuntary movements. Tremors or fasiculations while the patient is at rest suggest Parkinson's disease; their occurrence during motion suggests postural tremor. Determine muscle bulk, which is classified as normal, atrophy, hypertrophy, or pseudotrophy (bulk without strength, as in muscular dystrophy). Unilateral hand atrophy suggests median or ulnar nerve paralysis. Check tone by moving a relaxed limb through a range of motion. Describe any flaccidity or rigidity and then examine muscle strength, starting with grip strength and continuing through all limbs. Again note any asymmetry (the patient's dominant side should be slightly stronger). Observe the patient's gait and have him walk a straight line (heel to toe). Any ataxia suggests cerebellar disease, loss of position sense, or intoxication. Also have the patient walk on his toes, then heels; hop on each foot; and then do a shallow knee bend.

Perform a Romberg test (have him stand with his feet together and eyes closed for 20 to 30 seconds). Any excessive sway (a positive Romberg test) suggests ataxia from loss of position sense, whereas an inability to maintain balance with eyes open represents cerebellar ataxia. Ask the patient to hold his arms straight out in front with his palms up and eyes closed. Pronation suggests mild hemiparesis; drifting sideways or upward suggests loss of positional sense. Ask your patient to perform various rapid, alternating movements and observe for smoothness, speed, and rhythm. The dominant side should perform best, and any slow, irregular, or clumsy movements suggest cerebellar or extrapyramidal disease. Have your patient touch his thumb rapidly with the tip of the index finger, place his hand on his thigh and rapidly alternate from palm up to down, and assess for point-to-point testing (touch his nose, then your index finger several times rapidly or, for the legs, have him touch heel to knee, then run it down the shin).

Any jerking, difficulty in performing the task, or tremors suggest cerebellar disease. For position testing, have the patient perform the leg test with his eyes closed.

Evaluate the sensory system by testing sensations of pain, light touch, temperature, position, vibration, and discrimination. Compare responses bilaterally and from distal to proximal; then associate any deficit discovered with the dermatome it represents. Test superficial and deep tendon reflexes and note a dulled (cord or lower neuron damage) or hyperactive response (upper neuron disease).

Cranial nerves   pp. 146–154

CN-I is checked by evaluating the ability to sense odors in each nostril.

CN-II is checked by testing for visual acuity and field of view.

CN-III is checked by examining pupillary direct and consensual response.

CN-III, IV, and VI are checked by testing for smooth and unrestricted extraocular motion.

CN-V is checked by testing the masseter muscle strength and sensation on the forehead, cheek, chin, and cornea.

CN-VII is checked by examining the patient's face during conversations, looking for any asymmetry, eyelid droop, or abnormal movements.

CN-VIII is checked by evaluating for hearing and balance (with his eyes closed).

CN-IX and X are checked by evaluating speech, swallowing, saying "aaahhh," and the gag reflex.

©2013 Pearson Education, Inc.
Paramedic Care: Principles & Practice, Vol. 3, 4th Ed.

CN-XI is checked by testing trapezius and sternocleidomastoid muscles at rest and by evaluating head turning and shoulder raising.

CN-XII is checked by evaluating speech and having the patient extend his tongue outward.

Any deviation from a normally expected response is a reason to suspect a cranial nerve injury.

10. **Given a variety of scenarios, perform reassessment according to the patient's condition.** pp. 155–158

For stable patients, reassess every 15 minutes, and for unstable patients reassess every 5 minutes. Compare your findings to the baseline findings and note any trends. Include reassessment of the mental status, airway, breathing, circulation, skin condition, vital signs, focused assessments, and effects of interventions. Be sure to devise transport priorities and management plans as a patient's status changes.

11. **Adapt physical examination techniques to patients of all ages.** p. 71

Success in examining pediatric patients depends on familiarity with differences in anatomy and physiology, including differences in vital sign values, as well as understanding the developmental characteristics of children at all ages. Understand the reaction of children to strangers and the need to keep the family involved. Use age-appropriate language and place yourself at the patient's eye level.

Case Study Review

Reread the case study on pages 65 and 66 in Paramedic Care: Patient Assessment *before reading the following discussion.*

This case study clearly shows the benefit of a planned and well-directed physical examination of a patient with nonspecific signs and symptoms of disease. Here, Dale and Pam use the assessment to search out the possible causes, then converge, through specific signs and symptoms, on the patient's problem, which is their field diagnosis.

Matt and Ron arrive to care for a patient with very confusing and nonspecific signs and symptoms of illness. They and their patient, Mr. Dalton, count heavily on the comprehensive physical assessment to help sort out what might be wrong. A case like this is one of the few times you, as a paramedic, will employ most of the elements of a complete and detailed physical exam. More frequently, you will quickly identify the likely causes of your patient's chief complaint and presenting signs and symptoms—a differential diagnosis. Then you will focus your assessment on evaluating the presenting signs and symptoms and looking for those commonly associated with the diseases you suspect. This information then helps you rule out or support a problem, arriving at a single suspected problem—the field diagnosis.

Matt and Ron perform a quick primary survey to evaluate Mr. Dalton's mental status and ABCs. His first few words demonstrate that he is conscious and alert, and his airway and breathing are more than adequate. His mental status suggests his brain is being well perfused, and a quick pulse check confirms good circulation. With the elements of the primary survey complete, Matt and Ron move to the focused history and physical exam without a clear idea of what might be affecting Mr. Dalton.

Mr. Dalton's presentation is nonspecific to a particular medical problem; therefore, they must use the focused history and physical exam to investigate his physical and mental state more carefully. Elements of the patient history begin to direct their investigation toward a vascular problem: a history of coronary artery disease, hypertension, and the use of certain medications—nitroglycerin, aspirin, and digoxin. (Through his training and experience, Matt knows that nitroglycerin is given to reduce the demands on a heart with limited perfusion, that aspirin is used to reduce the risk of clot development, and that digoxin is often given for atrial fibrillation, which is frequently associated with pulmonary and cerebral emboli.) Added to the physical assessment finding—general weakness and an unstable walk and stance—what Matt and Ron learn suggests a motor or neurologic problem.

The team takes a quick set of vital signs that reveal only an abnormally high blood pressure, which is consistent with the history of hypertension. Matt performs the elements of the general survey and examines Mr. Dalton's appearance, level of consciousness, signs of distress, state of health, vital statistics, sexual development, skin color and lesions, posture, gait and motor activity, dress, grooming and personal hygiene, body or breath odor, and facial expression. They reveal a patient in generally good health with an appropriate affect. The only noted problem is one of coordinated walking (gait). The detailed physical exam reflects spasms at the outer reaches of left lateral eye movement, termed nystagmus. This, coupled with the gait problem, suggests a neurologic problem, for which Dale begins a complete neurologic exam.

Matt investigates posture, balance, reflexes, and coordination. Clearly, Mr. Dalton is slumped to the left side. Matt finds balance problems with Mr. Dalton, who drifts to the left when his eyes are closed. His reflexes are normal, at least for a 70-year-old man. His complaint about buttoning his shirt suggests a coordination problem, which Matt investigates further. He employs a few repetitive action exercises (thumb touch, shin touch, and palm-up/palm-down to thigh), which reveal a clear neurologic deficit on Mr. Dalton's left side.

Because of the left-sided slumping, nystagmus, and impaired coordination, Matt concludes that this is a cerebellar problem, most likely resulting from an arterial blockage. This is supported by both the history of earlier, less significant events (possibly transient ischemic events and an evolving stroke) and the vascular disease history discovered earlier. Note that motor and sensory function are controlled by the contralateral side of the brain (cerebral injury) and coordination is controlled by the ipsilateral cerebellum. In this scenario, Matt and Ron would also be likely to apply the cardiac monitor and evaluate the ECG for dysrhythmia. They might also auscultate the carotid arteries for bruit, suggestive of vascular disease that may be the origin of an embolus. In some EMS systems, stroke patients may be given clot-busting drugs, such as TPA or streptokinase, to dissolve blockage and reduce the effects of the infarct. In such a system, Matt and Ron may have a series of questions to ask of Mr. Dalton, to rule out the risk of internal hemorrhage, to help specifically identify the type of stroke or cerebrovascular accident, and to reduce the time from infarct to medication.

Content Self-Evaluation

MULTIPLE CHOICE

_____ 1. Of the physical examination techniques used in prehospital care, which is the LEAST invasive?
    A. Inspection   **D.** Percussion
    B. Auscultation   **E.** C and D
    C. Palpation

_____ 2. "Crackles" would be found using which of the following assessment techniques?
    A. Palpation   **D.** Percussion
    B. Auscultation   **E.** None of the above
    C. Inspection

_____ 3. "Tenderness" would be discovered using which of the following assessment techniques?
    A. Palpation   **D.** Percussion
    B. Auscultation   **E.** None of the above
    C. Inspection

_____ 4. Which of the following techniques should be performed first during the physical examination?
    A. Palpation   **D.** Percussion
    B. Auscultation   **E.** None of the above
    C. Inspection

_____ 5. Which part of the hands and fingers is best suited to evaluate tissue consistency?
    A. Tips of the fingers   **D.** Back of the hands or fingers
    B. Pads of the fingers   **E.** None of the above
    C. Palm of the hand

_____ 6. Which part of the hands and fingers is best suited to evaluate vibration?
    A. Tips of the fingers   **D.** Back of the hands or fingers
    B. Pads of the fingers   **E.** None of the above
    C. Palm of the hand

©2013 Pearson Education, Inc.
Paramedic Care: Principles & Practice, Vol. 3, 4th Ed.

_____ **7.** Noticing areas of warmth during palpation might reflect an injury before significant edema and discoloration develop.
   A. True
   B. False

_____ **8.** The booming sound produced by percussing an air-filled region is
   A. hyperresonance.   **D.** flat.
   B. dull.   **E.** none of the above.
   C. resonance.

_____ **9.** The only region where you perform auscultation as other than the last step of assessment is the
   A. anterior thorax.   **D.** peripheral arteries.
   B. neck.   **E.** posterior thorax.
   C. abdomen.

_____ **10.** A heart rate above 100 beats per minute is known as
   A. bradycardia.   **D.** tachypnea.
   B. tachycardia.   **E.** bradypnea.
   C. hypercardia.

_____ **11.** One likely cause of bradycardia is
   A. fever.   **D.** fear.
   B. pain.   **E.** blood loss.
   C. parasympathetic stimulation.

_____ **12.** Which of the following is NOT an aspect of pulse evaluation?
   A. Volume   **D.** Rate
   B. Rhythm   **E.** None of the above
   C. Quality

_____ **13.** Normal exhalation is
   A. an active process involving accessory muscles.
   B. an active process involving the diaphragm and intercostal muscles.
   C. active in its early stages and passive in later stages.
   D. passive in its early stages and active in later stages.
   E. a passive process.

_____ **14.** For a patient with an airway obstruction, exhalation is likely to be
   A. an active process involving accessory muscles.
   B. an active process involving only the diaphragm and intercostal muscles.
   C. active in its early stages and passive in later stages.
   D. passive in its early stages and active in later stages.
   E. a passive process.

_____ **15.** The amount of air a patient moves into and out of his lungs in one breath is the
   A. normal volume.   **D.** tidal volume.
   B. respiratory volume.   **E.** minute volume.
   C. residual volume.

_____ **16.** The pressure of the blood within the blood vessels while the ventricles are relaxing is the
   A. Korotkoff blood pressure.   **D.** asystolic blood pressure.
   B. systolic blood pressure.   **E.** atrial blood pressure.
   C. diastolic blood pressure.

_____ **17.** The diastolic blood pressure represents a measure of
   A. systemic vascular resistance.
   B. the cardiac output.
   C. the viscosity of the blood.
   D. the strength of ventricular contraction.
   E. relative blood volume.

18. Which of the following could influence a patient's blood pressure?
    A. Anxiety
    B. Position (lying, sitting, standing)
    C. Recent smoking
    D. Eating
    E. All of the above

19. Generally, hypertension in a healthy adult is any blood pressure higher than
    A. 120/80.
    B. 140/90.
    C. 160/90.
    D. 180/100.
    E. 200/100.

20. What is the pulse pressure in a patient with the following vital signs: pulse 82 and strong; respirations 14 and full; and blood pressure 144/96?
    A. 14
    B. 40
    C. 48
    D. 96
    E. 120

21. When testing orthostatic vital signs, what vital sign change is the most sensitive positive sign of hypovolemia?
    A. Blood pressure drops by 10 to 20 mmHg
    B. Blood pressure rises by 10 to 20 mmHg
    C. Pulse rate drops by 10 to 20 beats per minute
    D. Pulse rate rises by 10 to 20 beats per minute
    E. Either A or D

22. Hyperthermia can result from all of the following EXCEPT
    A. high environmental temperatures.
    B. infections.
    C. reduced metabolic activity.
    D. drugs.
    E. increases in metabolic activity.

23. What technique of stethoscope use best transmits low-pitched sound to the ear?
    A. Light pressure on the diaphragm
    B. Firm pressure on the diaphragm
    C. Moderate pressure on the bell
    D. Light pressure on the bell
    E. Strong pressure on the bell

24. The bell of a stethoscope is best for listening to the sounds of
    A. blood vessel bruits.
    B. the blood pressure.
    C. the heart.
    D. the lung.
    E. none of the above.

25. Which of the following is NOT a characteristic of a good stethoscope?
    A. Thick, heavy tubing
    B. Long tubing (70 to 100 cm)
    C. Snug-fitting earpieces
    D. A bell with a rubber-ring edge
    E. All of the above

26. Generally, each narrow line on a sphygmomanometer represents what pressure difference?
    A. 1 mmHg
    B. 2 mmHg
    C. 4 mmHg
    D. 5 mmHg
    E. 10 mmHg

27. If a patient has a regular and strong pulse, you should determine the pulse rate by assessing the number of beats in
    A. 2 minutes and dividing by 2.
    B. 3 minutes.
    C. 30 seconds and multiplying by 2.
    D. 15 seconds and multiplying by 4.
    E. 10 seconds and multiplying by 5.

28. Use of which of the following pulse points is recommended with a small child?
    A. Radial
    B. Brachial
    C. Carotid
    D. Popliteal
    E. Dorsalis pedis

©2013 Pearson Education, Inc.
Paramedic Care: Principles & Practice, Vol. 3, 4th Ed.

_____ **29.** It is important to attempt to evaluate your patient's respiratory rate and volume without his being aware of it.
  A. True
  B. False

_____ **30.** The proper position of the patient's arm when taking the blood pressure is
  A. arm slightly flexed.
  B. palm up.
  C. fingers relaxed.
  D. clothing removed from the upper arm.
  E. all of the above.

_____ **31.** The sphygmomanometer should be inflated to what level beyond the point at which the patient's radial pulse disappears?
  A. 10 mmHg
  B. 20 mmHg
  C. 30 mmHg
  D. 40 mmHg
  E. Between B and C

_____ **32.** The first blood pressure reading is the systolic blood pressure, indicated by the early deflections of the sphygmomanometer needle.
  A. True
  B. False

_____ **33.** When using an oral glass thermometer, it should be left in the mouth for what period of time?
  A. 30 to 45 seconds
  B. 30 to 60 seconds
  C. 1 to 2 minutes
  D. 2 minutes
  E. 3 to 4 minutes

_____ **34.** Pale skin is LEAST likely to be caused by which of the following?
  A. Increased deoxyhemoglobin
  B. A cold environment
  C. Shock compensation
  D. Anemia
  E. Hypovolemic shock

_____ **35.** Which of the following skin discolorations represents a yellow hue?
  A. Cyanosis
  B. Jaundice
  C. Eccyhmosis
  D. Erythema
  E. Pallor

_____ **36.** A heavy scaling of the skin under the hair is
  A. dandruff.
  B. nits.
  C. seborrheic dermatitis.
  D. psoriasis.
  E. none of the above.

_____ **37.** With age, the toenails are likely to become
  A. hard.
  B. thick.
  C. brittle.
  D. yellowish.
  E. all of the above.

_____ **38.** The bluish discoloration around the orbits of the eyes, suggestive of a basilar skull fracture, is called
  A. racoon eyes.
  B. Battle's sign.
  C. periorbital ecchymosis.
  D. retroauricular ecchymosis.
  E. either A or C.

_____ **39.** The cranial nerves that control eye movement are
  A. I, II, and III.
  B. II, III, and IV.
  C. III, IV, and VI.
  D. II, VI, and VII.
  E. V, VI, and VIII.

40. The muscular and colored portion of the eye that constricts and dilates to regulate light falling on the retinal surface is the
   A. retina.
   B. pupil.
   C. conjunctiva.
   D. iris.
   E. lens.

41. The characteristic of the unaffected eye responding to stimuli in the affected eye is
   A. consensual response.
   B. direct response.
   C. simultaneous response.
   D. ipsilateral response.
   E. none of the above.

42. About 20 percent of the population has a noticeable difference in the size of the pupils, a condition called
   A. hyphema.
   B. anisocoria.
   C. glaucoma.
   D. hypopyon.
   E. none of the above.

43. The ear provides what important body function beyond hearing?
   A. Equalization of pressure during yawning
   B. Vibration sensation
   C. Balance and head position sense
   D. Equalization of body and outside pressure
   E. All of the above except B

44. Otorrhea is a discharge from the ear that may contain
   A. pus.
   B. mucus.
   C. blood.
   D. cerebrospinal fluid.
   E. all of the above.

45. The term for a common nosebleed is
   A. epistaxis.
   B. otorrhea.
   C. rhinorrhea.
   D. rhinitis.
   E. none of the above.

46. The most superior and prominent airway structure in the neck is the
   A. cricoid cartilage.
   B. thyroid cartilage.
   C. tracheal ring.
   D. thyroid gland.
   E. jugular vein.

47. The layer of tissue that covers the interior of the chest wall and helps ensure that the lungs move with the thorax is the
   A. visceral pleura.
   B. parietal pleura.
   C. pertioneum.
   D. pulmonary pleura.
   E. perineum.

48. A likely location to notice retraction during forced inspiration is
   A. the suprasternal notch.
   B. the intercostal spaces.
   C. the supraclavicular space.
   D. all of the above.
   E. none of the above.

49. The type of motion associated with a free segment of the chest where the segment moves opposite to the rest of the chest during breathing is
   A. symbiotic.
   B. paradoxical.
   C. antagonistic.
   D. retractive.
   E. traumatic.

50. During the palpation of the chest, you should feel for which of the following?
   A. Tenderness
   B. Deformities
   C. Depressions
   D. Asymmetry
   E. All of the above

_____ **51.** During the check for chest excursion, the distance between your thumbs should increase by what amount during the patient's inspiration?
  - **A.** 2 cm
  - **B.** 3 to 5 cm
  - **C.** 5 to 6 cm
  - **D.** 10 to 12 cm
  - **E.** 0 cm

_____ **52.** Increased tactile fremitus suggests which of the following conditions?
  - **A.** Pneumonia
  - **B.** Pneumothorax
  - **C.** Pleural effusion
  - **D.** Emphysema
  - **E.** All of the above

_____ **53.** Which condition is most likely to cause an area of the lung that is dull to percussion?
  - **A.** Pneumothorax
  - **B.** Tension pneumothorax
  - **C.** Hemothorax
  - **D.** Pericardial tamponade
  - **E.** Friction rubs

_____ **54.** Light popping, nonmusical sounds heard in the chest during inspiration are known as
  - **A.** rhonchi.
  - **B.** stridor.
  - **C.** crackles.
  - **D.** wheezes.
  - **E.** none of the above.

_____ **55.** Hearing words transmitted clearly as you auscultate the chest with the stethoscope is a normal finding called bronchophony.
  - **A.** True
  - **B.** False

_____ **56.** The point of maximal impulse (PMI) in the adult is usually located at the
  - **A.** 3rd costal cartilage, close to the sternum.
  - **B.** 3rd intercostal space, just left of the sternum.
  - **C.** 5th intercostal space, just right of the sternum.
  - **D.** 5th intercostal space, near the midclavicular line.
  - **E.** 8th intercostal space, near the midclavicular line.

_____ **57.** Which listing represents the valves of the heart in order as blood flows through them from the vena cavae?
  - **A.** Tricuspid, pulmonic, mitral, aortic
  - **B.** Mitral, aortic, tricuspid, pulmonic
  - **C.** Pulmonic, tricuspid, aortic, mitral
  - **D.** Aortic, tricuspid, pulmonic, mitral
  - **E.** Tricuspid, aortic, mitral, pulmonic

_____ **58.** The "lub" of the heart sounds represents which event of the cardiac cycle?
  - **A.** Ejection of blood from the ventricles
  - **B.** Ventricular contraction
  - **C.** Ventricular filling
  - **D.** Closing of the aortic and pulmonic valves
  - **E.** Closing of the tricuspid and mitral valves

_____ **59.** Which of the following elements does NOT affect cardiac output?
  - **A.** Heart rate
  - **B.** Cardiac preload
  - **C.** Contractile force
  - **D.** Hematocrit
  - **E.** Peripheral vascular resistance

_____ **60.** Which of the following does NOT inhibit venous return to the heart?
  - **A.** Peripheral vascular resistance
  - **B.** Hypovolemia
  - **C.** Tension pneumothorax
  - **D.** Cardiac tamponade
  - **E.** Congestive heart failure

_____ **61.** Which abdominal organ is found in all four quadrants?
  - **A.** Stomach
  - **B.** Liver
  - **C.** Large intestine
  - **D.** Pancreas
  - **E.** Spleen

_____ 62. An eccyhmotic discoloration over the umbilicus is
- **A.** Grey Turner's sign.
- **B.** borborygmi.
- **C.** Hering-Breuer's sign.
- **D.** Cullen's sign.
- **E.** none of the above.

_____ 63. Auscultation of high-pitched gurgles and clicks every 5 to 15 seconds in the abdomen indicates
- **A.** borborygmi.
- **B.** increased bowel motility.
- **C.** absent bowel sounds.
- **D.** normal bowel sounds.
- **E.** ascites.

_____ 64. The fleshy folds that cover the vagina are the
- **A.** labia.
- **B.** clitoris.
- **C.** mons pubis.
- **D.** perineum.
- **E.** menarche.

_____ 65. The sound or feeling caused by unlubricated bone ends rubbing together is
- **A.** palpable fremitus.
- **B.** crepitus.
- **C.** bruit.
- **D.** friction rub.
- **E.** the pooh-pooh sign.

_____ 66. The type of movement permitted between the phalanges is
- **A.** abduction/adduction.
- **B.** rotation.
- **C.** flexion/extension.
- **D.** supination/pronation.
- **E.** both C and D.

_____ 67. Carpal tunnel syndrome involves which nerve?
- **A.** Brachial
- **B.** Median
- **C.** Radial
- **D.** Ulnar
- **E.** Olecranon

_____ 68. The type of movement permitted between the radius, ulna, and humerus is
- **A.** abduction/adduction.
- **B.** rotation.
- **C.** flexion/extension.
- **D.** supination/pronation.
- **E.** both C and D.

_____ 69. The joint that has the greatest range of motion of any joint in the human body is the
- **A.** shoulder.
- **B.** wrist.
- **C.** hip.
- **D.** elbow.
- **E.** ankle.

_____ 70. A major muscle of the calf is the
- **A.** bicep.
- **B.** tricep.
- **C.** gastrocnemius.
- **D.** hamstring.
- **E.** gracilis anterior.

_____ 71. The knee joint involves all of the following bones EXCEPT the
- **A.** femur.
- **B.** patella.
- **C.** tibia.
- **D.** fibula.
- **E.** all of the above.

_____ 72. The type of motion permitted by the knee joint is
- **A.** flexion/extension.
- **B.** adduction/abduction.
- **C.** inversion/eversion.
- **D.** limited rotation.
- **E.** both A and D.

_____ 73. Which region of the spine is most mobile?
- **A.** Cervical
- **B.** Thoracic
- **C.** Lumbar
- **D.** Sacral
- **E.** Coccygeal

74. The mid and lower cervical spine permits which type of movement?
  A. Flexion
  B. Extension
  C. Lateral bending
  D. Rotation
  E. All of the above

75. A lateral curvature of the spine is
  A. lordosis.
  B. scoliosis.
  C. kyphosis.
  D. spina bifida.
  E. none of the above.

76. Tenderness at a vertebral process and in the surrounding musculature of the lumbar spine is most likely due to
  A. vertebral process fracture.
  B. ligamentous injury.
  C. paravertebral muscular spasm.
  D. herniated intervertebral disk.
  E. none of the above.

77. A normal pulse quality would be reported as
  A. 0.
  B. 1+.
  C. 2+.
  D. 3+.
  E. 4+.

78. Which of the following is NOT a sign of proximal arterial occlusion?
  A. Thrills
  B. Pulse deficit
  C. Cold limb
  D. Poor color in the fingertips
  E. Slow capillary refill

79. Pitting edema that depresses 1/2 to 1 inch is reported as
  A. 0.
  B. 1+.
  C. 2+.
  D. 3+.
  E. 4+.

80. The pitting of edema will usually disappear within how many seconds after the release of pressure?
  A. 2
  B. 4
  C. 6
  D. 8
  E. 10

81. A complete neurologic exam includes which of the following areas?
  A. Cranial nerves
  B. Motor system
  C. Reflexes
  D. Sensory system
  E. All of the above

82. A patient who is drowsy but answers questions is considered to be
  A. lethargic.
  B. obtunded.
  C. stuporous.
  D. comatose.
  E. none of the above.

83. Normal speech is
  A. inflected.
  B. clear and strong.
  C. fluent and articulate.
  D. variable in volume.
  E. all of the above.

84. The term *dysphonia* refers to which of the following?
  A. Defective speech caused by motor deficits
  B. Voice changes due to vocal cord problems
  C. Defective language due to a neurologic problem
  D. Voice changes due to aging
  E. None of the above

85. The term *aphasia* refers to which of the following?
   A. Defective speech caused by motor deficits
   B. Voice changes due to vocal cord problems
   C. Defective language due to a neurologic problem
   D. Voice changes due to aging
   E. None of the above

86. Which of the following is one of the three basic grades of memory?
   A. Intermediate
   B. Verifiable
   C. Redux
   D. Remote
   E. Retrograde

87. A question about a patient's wife's birthday tests which of the following types of memory?
   A. Intermediate
   B. Verifiable
   C. Redux
   D. Remote
   E. Retrograde

88. During the test of extraoccular eye movement, you should trace which figure in front of your patient's eyes?
   A. An "X"
   B. An "H"
   C. A "1"
   D. A large "O"
   E. Any of the above

89. Stimulation for a blink by touching the eye's surface with fine cotton fibers tests which of the following?
   A. Corneal reflex
   B. Ptosis
   C. EOM
   D. The trigeminal nerve
   E. None of the above

90. When a person loses his sense of balance, which cranial nerve has most likely been injured?
   A. Equilibrial
   B. Glossopharyngeal
   C. Acoustic
   D. Vagus
   E. Accessory

91. Damage to CN-XII will cause the tongue to deviate in which manner?
   A. Downward
   B. Upward
   C. Toward the side of injury
   D. Away from the side of injury
   E. Furrowing and curving upward

92. The pyramidal pathway within the spinal cord mediates which of the following?
   A. Voluntary muscle control
   B. Involuntary muscle control
   C. Dermatome sensation
   D. Visceral sensation
   E. Vasoconstriction

93. Damage to the extrapyramidal pathways is likely to cause what type of presentation?
   A. Abnormal posture
   B. Abnormal gait
   C. Involuntary movement
   D. Increased muscle tone
   E. All of the above

94. The twitching of small muscle fibers is
   A. spasm.
   B. tics.
   C. tremors.
   D. fasciculations.
   E. atrophy.

95. In cases of muscular dystrophy, the patient's muscles
   A. increase in size.
   B. decrease in size.
   C. increase in strength.
   D. decrease in strength.
   E. both A and D.

©2013 Pearson Education, Inc.
Paramedic Care: Principles & Practice, Vol. 3, 4th Ed.

_____ 96. During your testing of a patient's muscle strength, you notice one side to be slightly stronger than the other. This is a normal finding.
   A. True
   B. False

_____ 97. Which of the following procedures describes the Romberg test? Have the patient
   A. walk heel-to-toe in a straight line.
   B. stand with eyes closed for 20 to 30 seconds.
   C. walk across the room and turn and walk back again.
   D. do a shallow knee bend on each leg in turn.
   E. walk first on his heels, then toes.

_____ 98. An area of skin innervated by a specific peripheral nerve root is a(n)
   A. afferent region.   D. dermatome.
   B. sensory topographic region.   E. both A and C.
   C. myotome.

_____ 99. The score on the muscle strength scale that describes a patient able to perform active movement against gravity is
   A. 5.   D. 2.
   B. 4.   E. 1.
   C. 3.

_____ 100. Babinski's response is positive when the sole of the foot is stroked and
   A. the big toe plantar flexes while other toes dorsiflex.
   B. the big toe plantar flexes while other toes fan out.
   C. the big toe dorsiflexes while other toes fan out.
   D. the big toe dorsiflexes while other toes plantar flex.
   E. all toes plantar flex.

_____ 101. In caring for the ill or injured child, it is important to be which of the following?
   A. Confident   D. Calm
   B. Direct   E. All of the above
   C. Honest

_____ 102. Children first recognize their parents' faces and voices at about what age?
   A. 2 months   D. 10 months
   B. 6 months   E. 1 year
   C. 8 months

_____ 103. Infants begin to sit up at about what age?
   A. 2 to 4 months   D. 10 months to 1 year
   B. 4 to 6 months   E. 1 year or later
   C. 6 to 8 months

_____ 104. The most difficult pediatric age group to assess is the
   A. infant.   D. school-age child.
   B. toddler.   E. adolescent.
   C. preschooler.

_____ 105. Which of the following groups is particularly distrusting of strangers?
   A. Infant   D. School-age child
   B. Toddler   E. Adolescent
   C. Preschooler

MATCHING

Match the cranial nerve number with its name and function by writing the appropriate numbers in the spaces provided.

Name

A. acoustic

B. optic

C. trochlear

D. abducens

E. accessory

F. glossopharyngeal

G. trigeminal

H. oculomotor

I. vagus

J. hypoglossal

K. facial

L. olfactory

Function

M. smell

N. posterior palate and pharynx motor control

O. trapezius and sternocleidomastoid motor control

P. sight

Q. tongue sensation

R. motor control of the tongue

S. motor control of the superior oblique muscles

T. anterior tongue sensation posterior pharynx motor control

U. lateral rectus muscle motor control

V. hearing and balance

W. eye movement and pupil constriction

X. forehead, cheek, and chin sensation

Cranial Nerve	Name	Function
106. I	_____	_____
107. II	_____	_____
108. III	_____	_____
109. IV	_____	_____
110. V	_____	_____
111. VI	_____	_____
112. VII	_____	_____
113. VIII	_____	_____
114. IX	_____	_____
115. X	_____	_____
116. XI	_____	_____
117. XII	_____	_____

Special Projects

Vital Signs

For each of the following vital signs, list the normal range of values and any other important considerations in their evaluation.

©2013 Pearson Education, Inc.
Paramedic Care: Principles & Practice, Vol. 3, 4th Ed.

Pulse:

_____

_____

_____

Respirations:

_____

_____

_____

_____

_____

_____

_____

Blood pressure:

_____

_____

_____

_____

_____

Temperature:

_____

_____

_____

_____

_____

Range of Motion Exercise

Identify the range of motion for each of the joints listed in the charts on the next page. Then fill in the rest by reviewing the text, pages 126 through 145.

It is not easy to remember and evaluate the range of motion for each joint of the extremities. To help you both remember the ranges of motion for each joint and assess the mobility of the patients you will treat, test your own joints for their ranges of motion against those from the text (and the following chart). Identify the joints where your movement exceeds or is less than the figures given in the book. Remember this difference. Then if you ever question how a patient's range of movements relates to the normal ranges, compare the patient's joint mobility to your own.

Physical Assessment—Personal Benchmarking

To perform the physical assessment of a patient, you will need to use the skills of inspection, palpation, auscultation, and percussion. You must not only master each of these skills but also learn to recognize normal and abnormal patient presentations. Often the distinction between normal and abnormal is very small and difficult to recognize without extensive experience. It is also difficult to maintain the ability to differentiate between normal and abnormal signs unless you practice the skill regularly. To help in skills maintenance, frequently use yourself as a physiological model upon which to practice assessment techniques and as a benchmark against which you can measure your patients' responses.

Upper Extremity

Joint	Flexion/Extension	Rotation	Other Motion
Wrist	_____/_____		(Medial/Lateral) _____/_____
Elbow	_____/_____		(Supination/Pronation) _____/_____
Shoulder	_____/_____	(Internal/External) _____/_____	(Abduction/Adduction) _____/_____

Lower Extremity

Joint	Flexion/Extension	Rotation	Other Motion
Ankle	(Dorsiflex/Plantar Flex) _____/_____		(Inversion/Eversion) _____/_____
Knee	_____/_____		
Hip	_____/_____	(External/Internal) _____/_____	(Abduction) _____/_____

Auscultation: You need a stethoscope for this exercise.

Apply the diaphragm of the stethoscope to the skin of your chest or abdomen. If you do not warm it first, you will be quite surprised at how cold it feels. Remember this as you are auscultating your patients' chests and abdomens.

Practice using the disk and diaphragm to ensure you know which setting sends bell sounds to your ears and which sends diaphragm sounds. Listen to the different sounds found at various locations around the chest and abdomen. Increase the pressure on the bell from gentle for low sounds to strong pressure for high-pitched sounds. You might also practice listening with the television on at various volume levels. This simulates background noise at the emergency scene and demonstrates how difficult it can be to assess breath, heart, and bowel sounds in the field.

Lung sounds: Review pages 107 through 109.

Listen to lung sounds in each of the five lung lobes. Remember that your patient's position will be reversed; his left lobes will be to your right. Take slow, deep breaths with your mouth open and listen for the faint noise of air moving through the small airways (normal or vesicular breath sounds). If you have a chance to auscultate your chest when you are experiencing the congestion of a cold, you may hear crackles or wheezes.

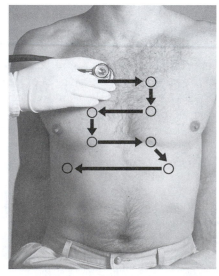

Then, auscultate the trachea at the suprasternal notch. Listen to the sounds; then move the diaphragm downward and laterally toward the lung fields. You will notice that the quality of the sounds changes as you move through the bronchial and bronchovesicular areas. Speak as you auscultate and notice how the speech sounds. It should be muffled, though you will hear it more clearly than when performing it on a patient, because some sound is transmitted through the bones of the face and skull in addition to the stethoscope.

Heart sounds: Review pages 114 through 116.

Review the accompanying illustration to identify the proper locations for auscultating the heart sounds. With each sound, increase the pressure on the bell from very light to heavy and appreciate the changing quality of the sounds. You might also palpate the carotid artery and then the radial pulse while auscultating to note the synchronization and delay between the sounds and pulse. Listen for the S1 and S2 sounds (the "lub-dub") of the normal heart.

Bowel sounds: Review pages 121 through 124.

Listen in each abdominal quadrant for at least 30 seconds to 1 minute with the diaphragm of your stethoscope. Listen very carefully in a very quiet environment because bowel sounds are difficult to decipher. Check your bowel sounds at various times during the day. They will likely be most frequent just before and right after a meal and before you go to sleep.

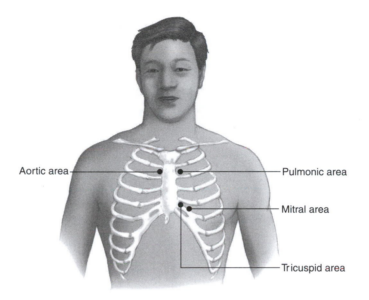

Aortic area — Pulmonic area — Mitral area — Tricuspid area

Physical Assessment—Personal Benchmarking

To perform the physical assessment of a patient, you will need to use the skills of inspection, palpation, auscultation, and percussion. You must not only master each of these skills but also learn to recognize normal and abnormal patient presentations. Often the distinction between normal and abnormal is very small and difficult to recognize without extensive experience. It is also difficult to maintain the ability to differentiate between normal and abnormal signs unless you practice the skill regularly. To help in skills maintenance, use yourself as a physiological model upon which to practice assessment techniques and as a benchmark against which you can measure your patients' responses.

Pulse location and evaluation: Review page 117.

Palpate each of the following arteries for the location, rate, and strength of pulsation.

   Radial—wrist, thumb side
   Ulnar—wrist, little finger side
   Brachial—medial aspect, just above the elbow
   Carotid—just lateral of the trachea (palpate both)
   Femoral—half the distance between the anterior iliac crest (the bone the belt sits on) and the symphysis
      pubis (just below the inguinal ligament)
   Popliteal—just behind and below the knee
   Posterior tibial—below the medial malleolus (ankle bone)
   Dorsalis pedis—on top of the foot

Locate each of these pulses on yourself, but realize that you are healthy and perfusing well. It is more difficult to find and evaluate these distal pulses on patients, especially the pulses on the lower extremities and those of patients with serious medical or trauma-induced problems. Remember to place the pads of your fingers lightly over the artery and increase the pressure until you feel the strongest impulse. Rate each pulse from 0 to 3+ (with 0 = absent, 1+ = weak or thready, 2+ = normal, 3+ = bounding). Practice finding and rating the pulses quickly. These skills will be invaluable when you assess your patients.

You might try counting a pulse in your arm or forearm while riding in a car. The vibration of travel makes the task much harder and simulates pulse evaluation in a moving ambulance. It might also be helpful to assess the pulses of friends and fellow emergency care workers to gain invaluable practice.

©2013 Pearson Education, Inc.
Paramedic Care: Principles & Practice, Vol. 3, 4th Ed.

Patient Monitoring Technology

Review of Chapter Objectives

After reading this chapter, you should be able to:

1. **Define key terms introduced in this chapter.**

   Knowing and being able to apply the key terms in each chapter is critical to understanding chapter concepts. Write the list of key terms. Then write the definition of each one in your own words. Check your understanding by confirming the definitions in the text glossary. Correct any misunderstandings. Create a study aid by writing each key term on the front of an index card and the definition on the back. Use the cards to quiz yourself, or to have someone quiz you.

2. **Describe the purpose, indications, procedure, normal findings, and limitations of the following patient monitoring technologies:**

   a. **Continuous ECG monitoring**   pp. 164–173

   Continuous electrocardiogram (ECG) monitoring is used to view a representation of the cardiac waveforms and associated segments and intervals to analyze the cardiac electrical rhythm. This then determines the pacemaker site and function, the spread of the electrical impulse through the cardiac conduction system, and the presence of any abnormal (ectopic) beats or arrhythmias. Continuous ECG monitoring provides important information about patients who are seriously ill, and who have complaints thought to be of cardiac origin. For routine cardiac monitoring, lead II is normally used. Place the monitor near the patient and turn it on and adjust the settings to view lead II. Place the electrodes according to the letters on them. Lead II uses the view from the right arm to the left leg, with a third electrode as a ground. View the dynamic ECG on the oscilloscope and, if desired, print a rhythm strip.

   The normal expected cardiac rhythm is normal sinus rhythm, which has specific characteristics as follows:

   - A positive P wave before every QRS complex
   - A PR interval from 0.12 to 0.20 seconds
   - A QRS complex of less than 0.12 seconds
   - The ST segment is at the isoelectric line
   - A positive, symmetrical T wave
   - Occasionally, a U wave
   - A rate from 60 to 100 per minute

Continuous ECG monitoring provides information about the electrical rhythm of the heart and gives some information about conduction; however, it only provides one view at a time of the electrical activity and does not give information about the mechanical function of the heart. Misinterpretation or interference can occur because of muscle tremors, shivering, patient movement, loose electrodes, 60-cycle electrical interference, and machine malfunction.

b. 12-lead ECG pp. 173–180

Twelve-lead ECGs provide 12 different views of the electrical activity of the heart, which is an important step in the assessment of patients with acute coronary syndrome (ACS). Twelve-lead ECGs are useful in detecting ST segment elevation myocardial infarction (STEMI), as well as a variety of other conditions that can affect the conduction of electrical impulses through the myocardium. This technology is used on patients with anginal equivalents, such as syncope, weakness, or dyspnea; stroke; pre-and post-cardioversion of stable patients; post-cardioversion of unstable patients; suspected electrolyte disturbances; overdoses; blunt chest trauma; dysrhythmias; respiratory failure; and heart failure.

To use the 12-lead ECG, you prepare the chest for adhesion of the electrodes, then place the four limb leads and six precordial (chest) leads. Make sure the patient lies still and then press the appropriate button to acquire the tracing. To look at the right side of the heart, add leads on the right chest that mirror those on the left chest. For a 15-lead ECG, add leads V4R, V8, and V9. For an 18-lead ECG, add V7 through V9 to view the posterior heart.

The normal appearance of each lead is based on the view of the myocardium and the direction of travel of the electrical flow with respect to each electrode. Leads I and aVL look at the left side of the heart vertically; leads II, III, and aVF look at the inferior surface of the heart; lead aVR looks at the right side of the heart vertically; leads V1 and V2 look at the right ventricle; leads V3 and V4 look at the intraventricluar septum and anterior aspect of the left ventricle; and leads V5 and V6 look at the anterior and lateral left ventricle. Like continuous ECG monitoring, a 12-lead ECG does not provide information about the mechanical function of the heart. A 12-lead ECG is a snapshot in time, and does not give continuous information, and mistakes in patient position, lead placement, and interpretation are common.

c. Pulse oximetry pp. 180–182

Pulse oximetry is a noninvasive method for determining the percentage of hemoglobin that is saturated, in order to give information about the patient's oxygenation. It is indicated for any patient in whom oxygenation may be a concern and as an adjunct to determine the effectiveness of treatments such as oxygen administration, ventilation, continuous positive airway pressure (CPAP), and bronchodilators.

A probe is connected to the monitoring device and attached to the patient's finger, toe, or earlobe (foot in infants). Make sure the pulse rate correlates with the pulse rate you obtained during vital signs. Observe the oxygen saturation reading on the device. Some devices, including those that measure carbon monoxide and methemoglobin, also measure total hemoglobin. At sea level, normal hemoglobin saturation is 96 to 100 percent.

Standard pulse oximetry cannot differentiate between hemoglobin that is saturated with oxygen and hemoglobin that is saturated with carbon monoxide and can give falsely high readings. It also cannot account for conditions in which the total amount of hemoglobin is reduced, such as in hemorrhage or shock. Although hemoglobin may be 100 percent saturated, it is the overall reduction in hemoglobin that results in tissue hypoxia in such patients. Incorrect sensor application and poor circulation can lead to inaccurate readings. Further, pulse oximetry cannot give information about other important measures of respiratory adequacy, such as carbon dioxide levels.

d. Capnography pp. 182–186

Capnography gives information about metabolism, circulation, and ventilation by measuring the amount of exhaled carbon dioxide. The amount of carbon dioxide in exhaled air is called end-tidal CO_2, or $ETCO_2$. $ETCO_2$ readings are an important part of the assessment of any critical patient to identify suspected problems with metabolic state, circulatory status, and ventilatory efficiency. It is used to confirm correct endotracheal tube placement and identify return of spontaneous circulation in cardiac arrest.

A sensor, either a simple colorimetric device that consists of litmus paper encased in plastic, or an electronic infrared sensor, is placed in the path of the patient's exhalation to detect CO_2. Normal $ETCO_2$ is between 35 and 45 mmHg, with an average normal of 38 mmHg. Levels above 45 mmHg

©2013 Pearson Education, Inc.
Paramedic Care: Principles & Practice, Vol. 3, 4th Ed.

indicate increased CO_2 production, decreased CO_2 elimination, or both. Readings below 35 mmHg indicate a decrease in CO_2 production, increase in CO_2 elimination, or both. Changes in $ETCO_2$ are reflective of changes in blood pH, which can seriously alter body functions.

Most limitations are associated with the use of the simple, disposable colorimetric devices, as their sensitivity and specificity are low. The devices only detect the presence of carbon dioxide and do not give an estimate of the amount present. The device can give inaccurate readings if exposed to gastric contents or used for a prolonged period of time.

e. **CO-oximetry**   pp. 187–189

Pulse CO-oximetry determines levels of oxygen (oxyhemoglobin), carbon monoxide (carboxyhemoglobin), and methemoglobin in the blood. The results allow you to rule in/rule out the presence of significant levels of carbon monoxide in the blood in order to properly treat patients with carbon monoxide poisoning and potentially identify patients with cyanide poisoning by eliminating carbon monoxide as a cause of signs and symptoms.

The device uses a probe like that described for pulse oximetry. The device has settings to read SpO_2, SpCO, and SpMet (methemoglobin). Readings over 15 to 20 percent COHb (carboxyhemoglobin) indicate mild carbon monoxide poisoning. As with pulse oximetry, limitations are related to the ability of the light sources to pass through tissue with adequate circulation.

f. **Methemoglobin monitoring**   pp. 189–192

Methemoglobin monitoring is used to detect methemoglobin, a form of hemoglobin that is not able to bind with oxygen. Methemoglobin is formed continuously as a result of the interaction between hemoglobin and oxygen, but normally the methemoglobin is converted back to hemoglobin at a rate that keeps the amount of methemoglobin low. Several drugs and toxins can increase the rate of methemoglobin production. Methemoglobinemia is uncommon, but some patients are at higher risk. Consider SpMet measurement in patients with uncorrectable cyanosis, patients receiving intravenous nitrates, or patients receiving treatment for cyanide poisoning with a three-part cyanide antidote kit.

The procedure is similar to that described for pulse oximetry and CO-oximetry, and a finding of 1 to 3 percent SpMet is considered normal. As with pulse oximetry and CO-oximetry, limitations are related to the ability of the light sources to pass through tissue with adequate circulation.

g. **Total hemoglobin**   p. 192

Hemoglobin is a protein that is carried on red blood cells. As hemoglobin levels decrease, the body's ability to oxygenate the body's tissues decreases. Total hemoglobin testing is used to measure the presence of anemia in any patient with excessive bleeding or dehydration, detect internal bleeding, triage the severity of a patient with signs of hypoperfusion, monitor the response to treatment of hyperperfusion, and document improvement or deterioration trends.

The procedure used to monitor total hemoglobin is the same as obtaining a patient's SpO_2, SpCO, and SpMet. A normal reading for an adult male should be between 14.0 and 17.4 g/dL, and an adult female level should be between 12.0 and 16.0 g/dL. The limitations to this procedure are the same as with pulse oximetry, CO-oximetry, and methemoglobin monitoring, where the accuracy of the score is dependent on the ability of the light sources to pass through tissue with adequate circulation.

h. **Glucometry**

Glucometry is used to identify hypoglycemic and hyperglycemic states, which helps in planning patient treatment. It should be used in patients with altered mental status and in patients who have a history of diabetes. Other patients who may benefit from glucometry include patients with seizures, head trauma, or stroke; pregnant patients or chronic alcoholics; patients with overdose of certain mediations; and patients with hepatitis or Addison's disease.

A drop of blood, generally obtained from a fingerstick, is placed on a test strip that has been inserted into an electronic blood glucometer device. The device gives a digital reading. A normal finding is considered to be 80 to 140 mg/dL. When performing this test you must be aware that poor preparation of the fingerstick site, expired test strips, or a poorly maintained or calibrated glucometer can give inaccurate readings.

i. **Basic blood chemistries (cardiac biomarkers, electrolytes, BNP, ABPs, serum lactate)**

Laboratory analysis of blood samples can provide information about patients presenting with vague complaints and can be used to confirm suspected conditions, such as myocardial infarction.

You may consider drawing blood for laboratory analysis when treatment you provide may alter the results of blood drawn later, or if the procedure will save time in getting laboratory results or reduce the number of needle sticks a patient may receive.

A special needle with a tube holder or a tube holder that adapts to an angiocath is used. Blood tubes slide into the holder where the rubber stopper at the top is punctured, allowing blood to fill the tubes. Tubes are filled in a particular order because of the substances contained in the tubes (red, blue, green, purple, gray). Fill tubes completely and gently agitate tubes containing anticoagulants or preservatives to mix. Properly label the tubes.

Normal findings depend upon the laboratory tests requested. Tests include cardiac biomarkers (creatne kinase, lactic dehydrogenase, myoglobin, tropinin, and B-natriuretic peptide) and electrolytes (such as sodium, potassium, chloride, bicarbonate, calcium, magnesium, phosphate, and serum lactate). Arterial blood gases require a different procedure to obtain blood from an arterial site, allowing measurement of the levels of oxygen, carbon dioxide, and bicarbonate, as well as allowing determination of the pH.

Limitations include the complications that can result from the venipuncture, and hemoconcentration and hemolysis of the blood sample.

Case Study Review

Reread the case study on page 163 in Paramedic Care: Patient Assessment; *then, read the following discussion. This case study identifies some of the uses of patient monitoring technology in the prehospital setting.*

Paramedic Rich Russell uses continuous cardiac monitoring, a 12-lead ECG, pulse oximetry with carbon monoxide and methemoglobin monitoring capabilities, capnography, and electronic noninvasive blood pressure monitoring to assist in the assessment of his patient, Paul Cuzins, who is experiencing upper abdominal discomfort and weakness. Using this technology, Rich is able to detect some ST segment elevation in the inferior ECG leads, indicating some ischemia. These technologies allow paramedics to better determine what is happening to a patient so the patient can receive more accurate and faster treatment.

Content Self-Evaluation

MULTIPLE CHOICE

_____ 1. The expected pacemaker of the heart is the
   A. sinoatrial node.
   B. right atrium.
   C. atrioventricular node.
   D. Bundle of His.
   E. Purkinje system.

_____ 2. The standard lead for continuous cardiac monitoring is lead
   A. aVR.
   B. aVF.
   C. I.
   D. II.
   E. III.

_____ 3. ECG lead II "reads" the flow of electricity through the heart from the
   A. right leg to the left arm.
   B. right arm to the left leg.
   C. right arm to the left arm.
   D. ground to the left arm.
   E. left arm to the left leg.

©2013 Pearson Education, Inc.
Paramedic Care: Principles & Practice, Vol. 3, 4th Ed.

4. On a standard ECG the light lines on the paper are 1 mm apart and represent _____ second.
   A. .02
   B. .04
   C. .06
   D. .12
   E. .20

5. In a lead II ECG, the first positive deflection in a normal rhythm is the _____ wave.
   A. Q
   B. R
   C. S
   D. P
   E. T

6. A lead II ECG is used to diagnose ST segment myocardial infarction.
   A. True
   B. False

7. Which of the following is characteristic of a pathological Q wave?
   A. It has a positive deflection.
   B. It is less than 25 mV.
   C. It is at least 1 mm wide.
   D. It is less than one-third the amplitude of the R wave in the same lead.
   E. It follows the R wave instead of preceding it.

8. The ECG leads aVR, aVL, and aVF are _____ leads.
   A. unipolar
   B. bipolar
   C. precordial
   D. chest
   E. right-sided

9. A limitation of a standard 12-lead ECG is
   A. it cannot show conduction defects in the His-Purkinje system.
   B. it only shows positive deflections.
   C. the inability to see most problems with the left side of the heart.
   D. the inability to assess the ST segment.
   E. the inability to show most problems with the right ventricle and posterior left ventricle.

10. The primary purpose of prehospital 12-lead ECGs is best described as
    A. not yet known and still being studied.
    B. ruling out acute coronary syndrome.
    C. monitoring the cardiac rhythm.
    D. accurately diagnosing congestive heart failure.
    E. reducing the time it takes for patients with STEMI to receive reperfusion therapy.

11. When an oxygen molecule binds to a heme structure, the result is
    A. carboxyhemoglobin.
    B. oxyhemoglobin.
    C. deoxyhemoglobin.
    D. methemoglobin.
    E. ferric hemoglobin.

12. The tendency for hemoglobin to more readily release oxygen molecules in conditions of low pH is called the Bohr effect.
    A. True
    B. False

13. The minimum acceptable SpO$_2$ reading at sea level is _____ percent.
   A. 100
   B. 98
   C. 95
   D. 92
   E. 90

14. How is the majority of carbon dioxide carried in the blood?
   A. Dissolved in plasma
   B. Bound to hemoglobin
   C. In the form of bicarbonate
   D. As carbon and oxygen molecules
   E. Dissolved in the cytoplasm of red blood cells

15. Arterial blood is considered acidic when its pH drops below
   A. 7.47.
   B. 7.45.
   C. 7.40.
   D. 7.35.
   E. 7.31.

16. Which of the following is an acceptable ETCO$_2$ value?
   A. 29 mmHg
   B. 33 mmHg
   C. 38 mmHg
   D. 41 mmHg
   E. Both C and D

17. Colorimetric capnometry is more reliable than continuous waveform capnography.
   A. True
   B. False

18. Waveform capnography can be used to determine the return of spontaneous circulation in a patient in whom CPR is being performed.
   A. True
   B. False

19. The half-life of carbon monoxide is reduced by 50 percent through the administration of 100 percent oxygen.
   A. True
   B. False

20. Carboxyhemoglobin levels are fatal at _____ percent.
   A. <15
   B. 20 to 40
   C. 41 to 50
   D. 55
   E. >60

21. Which of the following situations would be a strong indication for monitoring a patient's methemoglobin level?
   A. To assess for return of spontaneous circulation in cardiac arrest
   B. Receiving intravenous nitrates
   C. To continuously monitor endotracheal tube placement
   D. Acute asthma
   E. Patients receiving prolonged 100 percent oxygen

22. It is possible to noninvasively determine a patient's hemoglobin level.
   A. True
   B. False

©2013 Pearson Education, Inc.
Paramedic Care: Principles & Practice, Vol. 3, 4th Ed.

_____ **23.** Insulin is produced by the _____ cells of the pancreas.
  A. alpha
  B. delta
  C. beta
  D. acini
  E. tau

_____ **24.** A blood glucose level above _____ mg/dL is considered hyperglycemic.
  A. 80
  B. 100
  C. 120
  D. 140
  E. 160

_____ **25.** Patients for whom blood glucose determination is recommended include which of the following?
  A. Known diabetics
  B. Patients with altered mental status
  C. Alcoholics
  D. Patients with hepatitis
  E. All of the above

_____ **26.** The order in which blood tubes are filled makes no difference in the accuracy of test results.
  A. True
  B. False

_____ **27.** Which of the following is a cardiac biomarker?
  A. Bicarbonate
  B. Serum lactate
  C. Phosphate
  D. Lactic dehydrogenase
  E. $PaCO_2$

_____ **28.** A reason for measuring serum lactate is that it is a sensitive indicator of
  A. hypoperfusion.
  B. edema.
  C. myocardial injury.
  D. kidney function.
  E. heart failure.

_____ **29.** A suggested use of abdominal ultrasound in the prehospital setting is to
  A. determine the gestational age of a fetus.
  B. detect abdominal aortic aneurysm.
  C. assess heart valve function.
  D. assess lung function.
  E. all of the above.

_____ **30.** Abdominal ultrasound is effective in detecting relatively small amounts of peritoneal fluid.
  A. True
  B. False

MATCHING

Write the letter of the heart surface in the space provided next to the ECG leads used to assess it. Letters may be used more than once.

A. intraventricular septum and anterior left ventricle

B. posterior left ventricle

C. left side of the heart in a vertical plane

D. inferior side of the heart

E. right ventricle

F. additional view of right heart

G. anterolateral left ventricle

_____ 31. aVL

_____ 32. I

_____ 33. II

_____ 34. III

_____ 35. aVF

_____ 36. V1

_____ 37. V2

_____ 38. V3

_____ 39. V4

_____ 40. V5

_____ 41. V6

_____ 42. V4R

_____ 43. V9

Special Project

Deciding When to Use Patient Monitoring Technology

For each technology below, write at least one indication for its use in prehospital care.

Continuous ECG monitoring

_____

12-lead ECG

_____

Pulse oximetry

_____

Capnography

_____

Glucometry

_____

©2013 Pearson Education, Inc.
Paramedic Care: Principles & Practice, Vol. 3, 4th Ed.

Chapter

7

Patient Assessment in the Field

Review of Chapter Objectives

After reading this chapter, you should be able to:

1. Define key terms introduced in this chapter.

Knowing and being able to apply the key terms in each chapter is critical to understanding chapter concepts. Write the list of key terms. Then write the definition of each one in your own words. Check your understanding by confirming the definitions in the text glossary. Correct any misunderstandings. Create a study aid by writing each key term on the front of an index card and the definition on the back. Use the cards to quiz yourself, or to have someone quiz you.

2. Adapt the scene size-up, primary assessment, patient history, secondary assessment, and use of monitoring technology to meet the needs of the following types of patients:

a. Major trauma patient   **pp. 209–216**

For major trauma patients you will conduct a scene size-up, primary assessment, and rapid secondary assessment on the scene, and then package your patient and begin transport. En route, you will obtain a full set of vital signs and continue secondary assessment by reevaluating the mechanism of injury and will reassess your patient and perform treatments. Major trauma patients include those with serious mechanisms of injury, such as a fall from 20 feet or higher (adult), automobile crash with intrusion >12 inches at the occupant site or >18 inches at any site, partial or complete ejection, death of a passenger in the same vehicle, vehicle telemetry data that suggests high risk of injury, pedestrian struck by a vehicle, motorcycle crashes >20 mph, and bicyclists who are thrown, run over, or impacted at >20 mph.

The rapid secondary assessment is designed to identify life-threatening conditions that were not found in the primary assessment. It is fast and systematic, but not a detailed physical exam that would reveal even the most minor injuries, and you must conduct it before your patient is packaged. Begin by reassessing the mental status using AVPU. Use the techniques of inspection, palpation, auscultation, and percussion, as needed, to examine the head, neck, chest, abdomen, pelvis, and extremities. Examine the posterior aspect of the body as you log roll the patient. Treat life-threatening injuries, such as significant hemorrahge, inadequate ventilation, and tension pneumothorax, as you find them.

When indicated, immobilize the patient on a long spine board, maintaining in-line stabilization of the head and neck.

Obtain a medical history en route.

Reassessment consists of checking the mental status, airway, breathing, circulation, and deterioration in any areas already identified as problems. Also check the skin condition, vital signs, aspects of the secondary assessment, and effects of interventions. Based on the comparison of reassessment findings to your baseline findings, reevaluate transport priorities and management plans.

b. **Minor trauma patient**   pp. 216–218

Minor trauma patients do not have a significant mechanism of injury and have isolated, not systemic, problems, such as laceration or sprain. Perform a scene size-up, then begin with a primary assessment to ensure that the patient is alert and has adequate airway, breathing, and circulation. Perform an evaluation of the isolated injury, obtain a set of vital signs, and take a medical history. Reassess during transport.

c. **Unresponsive medical patient**   pp. 222–223

The approach to an unresponsive medical patient bears some similarity to the assessment of a major trauma patient. You will complete a scene size-up, perform a primary assessment, and complete a rapid secondary assessment. Then, obtain baseline vital signs and determine the history from by-standers, family, friends, or medical identification devices. Perform any additional monitoring or testing, such as cardiac monitoring or glucometry, as needed. Expedite transport and reassess the patient every 5 minutes.

d. **Responsive medical patient**   pp. 218–222

With a responsive medical patient, the history takes precedence over the physical exam. The history will generally provide your field diagnosis, which you will confirm with physical exam findings. The secondary assessment is used to look for signs of medical complications, rather than injury, and is guided by the history. Depending on the patient's condition, some treatments may need to proceed simultaneously.

In the history, obtain the chief complaint, and explore this further using the mnemonic OPQST-ASPN. Ask about the past medical history and family/social history, and perform a review of systems. Once you have obtained the history, perform a focused physical exam based on information from the history. Reassess the patient during transport.

3. **Use a process of clinical reasoning to guide and interpret the findings of patient assessment in the field.**   pp. 225–227

Clinical decision making requires that you effectively analyze data and develop practical management plans. Steps in critical thinking include: form a concept, interpret the data, apply principles, evaluate results, and reflect on the case.

Begin by gathering information through your assessment process and form a concept of the patient and the scene. The concept will be refined as you collect more information, and the emerging concept will guide further collection of information. Compare your concept to your database of experience and knowledge to develop a field diagnosis. Devise a management plan that covers all contingencies, using the protocols, standing orders, and interventions at your disposal. When needed, consult with medical direction. Reassess your patient and the effects of your interventions. Revise your field diagnosis and treatment as needed. After the call, obtain feedback and reflect on the case. Compare your field diagnosis with the physician's diagnosis. Make every patient contact a learning experience.

Case Study Review

Reread the case study on page 206 in Paramedic Care: Patient Assessment; *then, read the following discussion.*

This case study gives you the opportunity quickly to identify and review the elements of the patient assessment process by presenting a responsive medical patient in obvious distress. The process involves the scene size-up, primary assessment, history, secondary assessment, and reassessment.

©2013 Pearson Education, Inc.
Paramedic Care: Principles & Practice, Vol. 3, 4th Ed.

EMS providers Courtney and Ron respond to a college campus for a severe allergic reaction. Their scene size-up reveals an 18-year-old woman in obvious distress with difficulty swallowing. The history provides important information that guides the next actions: the patient has a history of allergic reactions, was exposed to a possible allergen, and feels like she is having a more severe reaction than she has had in the past. The assessment focuses on areas important to the known history and reveals respiratory distress.

Courtney and Ron begin immediate interventions, which worked quickly. However, Courtney and Ron know that the patient's signs and symptoms may return and convince the patient to be transported. Courtney continues to reassess the patient en route and adjusts her treatments to the patient's condition.

Courtney and Ron received important feedback about their clinical reasoning process from the emergency department physician to allow them to continue to refine their knowledge and decision-making processes.

Content Self-Evaluation

MULTIPLE CHOICE

_____ 1. As a paramedic, you will usually select which components of the exam are applicable to specific patients, rather than performing all components of the exam.
   A. True
   B. False

_____ 2. Which component of the patient assessment process will be performed during patient transport, regardless of the patient's condition?
   A. Scene size-up
   B. Primary assessment
   C. Focused history and physical exam
   D. Detailed physical exam
   E. Reassessment

_____ 3. As you approach a patient, he does not appear to be responsive or breathing. The mnemonic that guides your next steps is
   A. ABC.
   B. OPQRST-ASPN.
   C. CAB.
   D. SAMPLE.
   E. AEIOU-TIPS.

_____ 4. The first step in patient assessment for all patients is
   A. primary assessment.
   B. initial assessment.
   C. secondary assessment.
   D. scene size-up.
   E. focused history and physical exam.

_____ 5. Initially determining priorities of care and transport is part of the
   A. scene size-up.
   B. primary assessment.
   C. secondary assessment.
   D. reassessment.
   E. focused assessment.

_____ 6. The focused history and physical exam are conducted differently for the four different categories of patients. Which of the following is NOT one of those categories?
   A. Responsive medical patient
   B. Unresponsive medical patient
   C. Pediatric patient with altered consciousness
   D. Minor trauma patient
   E. Major trauma patient

7. Which of the following is NOT a mechanism of injury that calls for rapid transport to the trauma center?
    A. Ejection from a vehicle
    B. Vehicle rollover
    C. Severe vehicle deformity in a high-speed crash
    D. Fall from less than 20 feet for an adult
    E. Bicycle collision with loss of consciousness

8. The initial decision to provide rapid transport of a patient to the trauma center is predicated upon either the mechanism of injury or the
    A. blood pressure reading.
    B. serious clinical findings.
    C. pulse oximetry reading.
    D. reassessment.
    E. none of the above.

9. Which of the following body regions is examined during the rapid trauma assessment?
    A. Head
    B. Neck
    C. Pelvis
    D. Thorax
    E. All of the above

10. Scalp wounds tend to bleed heavily because
    A. there is a lack of a protective vasospasm mechanism.
    B. the hair helps continue the blood loss.
    C. the close proximity of the skull permits blood to flow quickly outward.
    D. direct pressure is difficult to apply.
    E. both A and C.

11. Subcutaneous emphysema is best described as
    A. a grating sensation.
    B. air trapped under the skin.
    C. air leaking from the respiratory system.
    D. retraction of the tissues between the ribs.
    E. fluid accumulation just beneath the skin.

12. Suprasternal and intercostal retractions are caused by
    A. tension pneumothorax.
    B. subcutaneous emphysema.
    C. airway obstruction or restriction.
    D. flail chest.
    E. either B or D.

13. To ensure adequate air exchange for the patient with a flail chest, you should
    A. perform a needle decompression.
    B. assist ventilations with a BVM and oxygen.
    C. apply oxygen only.
    D. perform an endotracheal intubation.
    E. cover the wound with an occlusive dressing.

14. When assessing the pelvis for possible fracture, you should apply
    A. anterior pressure on the iliac crests.
    B. lateral pressure on the symphysis pubis.
    C. firm pressure on the lower abdomen.
    D. medial and posterior pressure on the iliac crests.
    E. pressure to move the hips to the flexed position.

15. Your finding that a patient is able to move a limb but the limb is cool, pale, and without a pulse is consistent with
    A. neurologic compromise.
    B. vascular compromise.
    C. both a vascular and a neurologic compromise.
    D. spinal injury.
    E. peripheral nerve root injury.

©2013 Pearson Education, Inc.
Paramedic Care: Principles & Practice, Vol. 3, 4th Ed.

_____ 16. The "A" of the SAMPLE history stands for
   A. alcohol consumption.
   B. adverse reactions.
   C. attitude.
   D. allergies.
   E. none of the above.

_____ 17. With a patient who has a crushing injury to his index finger received when it was caught in a closing door, which form of patient assessment would be most reasonable?
   A. The rapid trauma assessment and a focused history
   B. The rapid trauma assessment and a detailed history
   C. A focused history and a physical exam focused on the injury
   D. A detailed patient history and a physical exam focused on the injury
   E. A detailed physical exam

_____ 18. While gathering the history of a chest pain patient, you will likely
   A. attach a cardiac monitor.
   B. administer oxygen.
   C. take vital signs.
   D. start an IV, if appropriate.
   E. all of the above.

_____ 19. The pain or discomfort that caused the patient to call you to his side is called the
   A. presenting problem.
   B. differential diagnosis.
   C. field diagnosis.
   D. chief complaint.
   E. present illness.

_____ 20. A patient statement that "deep breathing makes my chest hurt" represents which element of the OPQRST-ASPN mnemonic for investigation of the chief complaint?
   A. O
   B. P
   C. R
   D. S
   E. PN

_____ 21. The jugular veins in a patient with normal cardiovascular function remain full or distended up to which of the following degrees of patient tilt?
   A. 15°
   B. 30°
   C. 45°
   D. 60°
   E. 90°

_____ 22. If you hear bilateral crackles on inspiration when auscultating a patient's chest, you should suspect
   A. congestive heart failure.
   B. bronchospasm.
   C. asthma.
   D. chronic obstructive pulmonary disease.
   E. all of the above.

_____ 23. In a patient who displays hyperresonance to percussion of the chest, you should suspect
   A. pleural effusion.
   B. pulmonary edema.
   C. pneumonia.
   D. emphysema.
   E. none of the above.

_____ 24. Examine a patient for unusual pulsation of the descending aorta
   A. just right of the umbilicus.
   B. just left of the umbilicus.
   C. along a line from the umbilicus to the middle symphysis pubis.
   D. just beneath the xiphoid process.
   E. anywhere in the abdomen.

_____ 25. Accumulation of fluid within the abdominal cavity is common in patients with
   A. hypovolemia.
   B. aortic aneurysm.
   C. emphysema.
   D. gastric ulcer disease.
   E. cirrhosis of the liver.

26. A patient in whom unequal pupils is a normal condition displays
   - A. Cullen's sign.
   - B. anisocoria.
   - C. consensual response.
   - D. accommodation.
   - E. Bell's palsy.

27. The type of patient most likely to receive the most comprehensive assessment is
   - A. the severe trauma patient.
   - B. the minor trauma patient.
   - C. the responsive medical patient.
   - D. the unresponsive medical patient.
   - E. both A and D.

28. Serial reassessments will facilitate
   - A. identifying trends in the patient's condition.
   - B. revision of the field diagnosis.
   - C. changes in the management plan.
   - D. documentation of the effects of interventions.
   - E. all of the above.

MATCHING

Write the letter of the step in the critical decision-making process in the space provided next to the emergency response action appropriate for that step.

- A. form a concept
- B. interpret the data
- C. apply the principles
- D. evaluate the results
- E. reflect on the case

_____ 29. Field diagnosis

_____ 30. Provide reassessment

_____ 31. Perform the focused physical exam

_____ 32. Pulse oximetry

_____ 33. Follow standing orders

_____ 34. Differential diagnosis

_____ 35. Assess ABCs

_____ 36. Employ protocols

_____ 37. Determine the initial vital signs

_____ 38. Determine if treatment is improving the patient's condition

_____ 39. Follow up on the patient's diagnosis

©2013 Pearson Education, Inc.
Paramedic Care: Principles & Practice, Vol. 3, 4th Ed.

Special Project

Clinical Reasoning Process

Summarize the five steps of the clinical reasoning process.

Form a concept

_____

Interpret the data

_____

Apply the principles

_____

Evaluate the results

_____

Reflect on the case

_____

PATIENT ASSESSMENT
Content Review
Content Self-Evaluation

Chapter 1: Scene Size-Up

____ 1. Which of the following are items you should inform dispatch of following your scene size-up, if necessary?
   A. The phone number at which you can be reached
   B. Whether the emergency is a medical or trauma problem
   C. What resources you need
   D. What actions you and your crew are taking
   E. All of the above except A

____ 2. Which of the following types of protective equipment must you use on every call that results in patient contact?
   A. Protective eyewear
   B. Latex or vinyl gloves
   C. Gown
   D. Face mask
   E. Both B and C

____ 3. Which of the following should you wear if you are going to perform advanced airway procedures?
   A. Latex or vinyl gloves and a gown
   B. Protective eyewear, a gown, and a face mask
   C. Latex or vinyl gloves, protective eyewear, and a face mask
   D. Protective eyewear and a gown
   E. Latex or vinyl gloves

____ 4. Which of the following criteria must be met in order for you to effectively handle scene safety issues?
   A. You must be properly trained.
   B. You must have the right equipment.
   C. You must have the right personal protective equipment.
   D. You must be willing to do whatever it takes to make the scene safe.
   E. A, B, and C.

____ 5. Which scenario has the LEAST likelihood of having multiple patients?
   A. Car vs. motorcycle collision
   B. Carbon monoxide poisoning in a home
   C. Car crash in which a child safety seat and toys are visible
   D. Fall from a roof
   E. Hazardous materials spill in a high school chemistry lab

____ 6. You should call for additional ambulances as soon as the scene size-up tells you there are multiple patients, regardless of how minor the injuries might be.
   A. True
   B. False

____ 7. Which of the following is determined by analysis of the mechanism of injury?
   A. Anatomical location of injuries
   B. Velocity of crash forces
   C. Direction of the crash forces
   D. Whether restraint systems were used
   E. All of the above

_____ 8. Which of the following sources of information can give you information about the nature of the illness on a medical call?
   A. The patient
   B. The patient's family
   C. Unusual odors
   D. Medications at the scene
   E. All of the above

Chapter 2: Primary Assessment

_____ 9. Which of the following is NOT part of the primary assessment?
   A. Developing a general impression of the seriousness of the patient's condition
   B. Providing manual motion restriction of the cervical spine, if needed
   C. Obtaining baseline vital signs
   D. Opening the airway, if needed
   E. Controlling major hemorrhage

_____ 10. At which point during the primary assessment should you manually stabilize the cervical spine, if indicated?
   A. Immediately, if the MOI suggests the potential for spinal injury
   B. Just before you attempt artificial ventilation
   C. After establishing an airway
   D. After checking the circulation
   E. After checking the mental status

_____ 11. All of the following may cause an altered mental status EXCEPT
   A. shock.
   B. diabetic emergency.
   C. stroke.
   D. exposure to toxins.
   E. activation of the "flight or fight" response.

_____ 12. Your patient flinches when you pinch his trapezius muscle, but does not respond to anything you say. He is categorized, according to the AVPU mnemonic, as
   A. A.
   B. V.
   C. P.
   D. U.
   E. AP.

_____ 13. Which of the following is NOT a cause of stridor?
   A. Respiratory infection
   B. Laryngeal edema
   C. Foreign body in the airway
   D. Swallowed foreign body
   E. Allergic reaction

_____ 14. Your patient was rescued after being trapped in an apartment fire. He has soot around his mouth and nose and stridor on inspiration. The procedure that is most likely to provide definitive airway control for this patient is
   A. suctioning.
   B. early endotracheal intubation.
   C. a surgical airway.
   D. an albuterol treatment.
   E. low-flow oxygen and avoiding agitation.

_____ 15. Which of the following describes a state of abnormally deep breathing?
   A. Hyperpnea
   B. Tachypnea
   C. Eupnea
   D. Bradypnea
   E. Hypopnea

©2013 Pearson Education, Inc.
Paramedic Care: Principles & Practice, Vol. 3, 4th Ed.

_____ 16. When a patient has a radial pulse, it suggests that the systolic blood pressure is at least
  A. 60 mmHg.   D. 100 mmHg.
  B. 70 mmHg.   E. 120 mmHg.
  C. 80 mmHg.

_____ 17. You have discovered an elderly man lying on the floor of his living room. His wife states that he was fine when she went to get a snack, but when she returned a few minutes later, he had collapsed on the floor. The patient does not respond to painful stimulus. Which is the best way of opening this patient's airway?
  A. Oropharyngeal airway maneuver   D. Triple airway maneuver
  B. Modified jaw-thrust maneuver   E. Needle cricothryroidotomy
  C. Head-tilt/chin-lift maneuver

_____ 18. Your patient is a 24-year-old woman suspected of taking a heroin overdose. She has a pulse, but is not breathing adequately. You should provide bag-valve-mask ventilations at a rate of _____ per minute.
  A. 6 to 8
  B. 8 to 10
  C. 10 to 12
  D. 12 to 16
  E. 16 to 20

_____ 19. If the heart rate of a 9-year-old child is above _____ per minute, you should suspect a problem with circulation.
  A. 110   D. 80
  B. 100   E. 70
  C. 90

_____ 20. In the primary assessment, you are trying to find all problems a patient may have.
  A. True.
  B. False.

Chapter 3: Therapeutic Communications

_____ 21. Which of the following is a good example of an open-ended question in the patient history?
  A. What is bothering you today?
  B. Do you take heart medication?
  C. Does your pain get worse when you move around?
  D. Are you nauseated?
  E. How old are you?

_____ 22. Which of the following is an example of a closed-ended question?
  A. What does your pain feel like?
  B. What were you doing when the pain started?
  C. Why did you call us today?
  D. Have you vomited today?
  E. How are you feeling?

_____ 23. Using a patient's first name is the best way to establish rapport with most patients.
  A. True
  B. False

_____ 24. A good way to be thorough in your history is to have a prearranged list of questions that you ask all patients.
  A. True
  B. False

_____ 25. The statement, "You say your abdomen doesn't hurt, but I notice you seem to be uncomfortable lying flat," illustrates a therapeutic communication process called
  A. empathy.
  B. confrontation.
  C. reflection.
  D. clarification.
  E. facilitation.

_____ 26. While transporting a patient who had initially given you a good history, she suddenly stops talking and answers you only by nodding, shaking her head, and shrugging her shoulders. The best approach for this patient is to
  A. stay calm and continue to assess her body language.
  B. tell her you can't be of much help if she continues to refuse to cooperate.
  C. terminate the interview immediately.
  D. stop talking to the patient.
  E. let her know her behavior is not acceptable.

_____ 27. If your patient begins to cry, you should encourage him to try to calm down and pull himself together.
  A. True
  B. False

Chapter 4: History Taking

_____ 28. In the majority of medical cases, what information provides the primary basis of a paramedic's field diagnosis?
  A. Chief complaint
  B. Index of suspicion
  C. Mechanism of injury
  D. Patient history
  E. Vital signs

_____ 29. The process of narrowing down a list of hypotheses about a patient's problem to a short list of the most likely causes is called
  A. developing an index of suspicion.
  B. identifying the mechanism of injury.
  C. developing a differential field diagnosis.
  D. performing a CAGE questionnaire.
  E. establishing the nature of the illness.

_____ 30. The chief complaint is the same thing as the nature of the illness.
  A. True
  B. False

_____ 31. Which documented statement below describes a palliating factor?
  A. Pain increases with movement.
  B. The pain is the same as the patient's last migraine headache.
  C. The patient has had diarrhea for three days.
  D. The patient becomes dizzy when he moves his head.
  E. Epigastric pain is relieved immediately after meals.

_____ 32. A patient tells you he called 911 because he developed chest pain. This statement is the patient's
  A. primary problem.
  B. chief complaint.
  C. nature of the illness.
  D. mechanism of injury.
  E. none of the above.

_____ 33. Your patient is complaining of chest pain, and you believe, based on the history and exam findings, the reason for the pain is acute coronary syndrome. Possible acute coronary syndrome is the patient's
  A. primary problem.
  B. chief complaint.
  C. nature of the illness.
  D. mechanism of injury.
  E. none of the above.

©2013 Pearson Education, Inc.
Paramedic Care: Principles & Practice, Vol. 3, 4th Ed.

_____ **34.** A list of a patient's medications is important because these medications can contribute to the current medical problem as a result of

A. overmedication.

B. undermedication.

C. allergic reaction.

D. untoward reaction.

E. all of the above.

_____ **35.** A patient who has smoked 14 packs of cigarettes a week for 20 years has a pack history of

A. 20 pack/years.

B. 14 pack/years.

C. 7 pack/years.

D. 40 pack/years.

E. 10 pack/years.

_____ **36.** While reviewing the patient history form provided to you when you picked up your patient at a physician's office, you note the documentation G2P1A0L1. From this you know that the patient

A. is currently pregnant and has one living child.

B. is currently pregnant and lost one child.

C. had one past pregnancy and one miscarriage.

D. had one normal pregnancy and one complicated pregnancy.

E. has had one pregnancy that resulted in twins.

_____ **37.** Which of the following provider characteristics is NOT part of effective clinical reasoning?

A. The ability to gather data

B. The ability to sort relevant from irrelevant data

C. A fund of knowledge about pathophysiology and expected normal findings

D. The ability to compare a patient's presentation with that of other patients you have seen

E. The ability to come to a definitive diagnosis for all patients

Chapter 5: Secondary Assessment

_____ **38.** The least invasive physical exam technique is

A. inspection.

B. auscultation.

C. palpation.

D. percussion.

E. C and D.

_____ **39.** Which assessment technique would you use to determine if crackles are present?

A. Palpation

B. Auscultation

C. Inspection

D. Percussion

E. None of the above

_____ **40.** Which assessment technique would you use to determine if the patient has tenderness?

A. Palpation

B. Auscultation

C. Inspection

D. Percussion

E. None of the above

_____ **41.** Palpation can help identify areas of injury before visible signs appear.

A. True

B. False

_____ **42.** Which term is used to describe the flat sound produced by percussing an area that contains fluid or solid structures?

A. Resonance

B. Dull

C. Hyperresonance

D. Flat

E. None of the above

_____ **43.** When the heart rate of an adult is greater than 100 per minute, you should recognize this finding as

A. bradycardia.

B. tachycardia.

C. hypercardia.

D. tachypnea.

E. bradypnea.

_____ 44. Which of the following is a cause of an abnormally slow heart rate?
   A. Fever
   B. Pain
   C. Parasympathetic stimulation
   D. Fear
   E. Blood loss

_____ 45. Which statement best describes physiologically normal exhalation?
   A. An active process involving accessory muscles
   B. An active process involving the diaphragm and intercostal muscles
   C. Active in its early stages and passive in later stages
   D. Passive in its early stages and active in later stages
   E. A passive process

_____ 46. _____ is the amount of air a person moves into and out of his lungs in one breath.
   A. Normal volume
   B. Respiratory volume
   C. Residual volume
   D. Tidal volume
   E. Minute volume

_____ 47. When the left ventricle is relaxed, the amount of pressure that remains in the blood vessels is the _____ blood pressure.
   A. Korotkoff
   B. systolic
   C. diastolic
   D. asystolic
   E. atrial

_____ 48. Stimuli that affect a person's blood pressure include
   A. anxiety.
   B. position (lying, sitting, standing).
   C. recent smoking.
   D. eating.
   E. all of the above.

_____ 49. A blood pressure greater than _____ mmHg in an adult is considered hypertension.
   A. 120/80
   B. 140/90
   C. 160/90
   D. 180/100
   E. 200/100

_____ 50. You have recorded vital signs in a patient while he was supine. Now, after he has been standing, you recheck his vital signs. Which of the following changes is the most sensitive sign that the patient is suffering from hypovolemia?
   A. Blood pressure drops by 10 to 20 mmHg
   B. Blood pressure rises by 10 to 20 mmHg
   C. Pulse rate drops by 10 to 20 beats per minute
   D. Pulse rate rises by 10 to 20 beats per minute
   E. Either A or D is correct

_____ 51. Which of the following is NOT a cause of abnormally high body temperature?
   A. High environmental temperatures
   B. Infections
   C. Reduced metabolic activity
   D. Drugs
   E. Increases in metabolic activity

_____ 52. Which sounds would be heard best using the bell of your stethoscope?
   A. Blood vessel bruits
   B. The blood pressure
   C. The heart
   D. The lung
   E. None of the above

_____ 53. When purchasing a stethoscope, you should look for one that has all of the following characteristics EXCEPT
   A. thick, heavy tubing.
   B. long tubing (70 to 100 cm).
   C. snug-fitting earpieces.
   D. a bell with a rubber-ring edge.
   E. all of the above

_____ 54. For patients with a regular pulse, you should assess the heart rate by counting the number of beats in
A. 2 minutes and dividing by 2.
B. 3 minutes.
C. 30 seconds and multiplying by 2.
D. 15 seconds and multiplying by 4.
E. 10 seconds and multiplying by 5.

_____ 55. When checking the pulse of a small child, the best place to do so is the _____ artery.
A. radial
B. brachial
C. carotid
D. popliteal
E. dorsalis pedis

_____ 56. Which statement describes the positioning of a patient's arm to obtain an accurate blood pressure?
A. Arm slightly flexed
B. Palm up
C. Fingers relaxed
D. Clothing removed from the upper arm
E. All of the above

_____ 57. When taking a blood pressure, inflate the cuff _____ beyond the point at which the radial pulse is last felt.
A. 10 mmHg
B. 20 mmHg
C. 30 mmHg
D. 40 mmHg
E. between B and C

_____ 58. Which of the following would NOT adequately explain pale skin color?
A. Increased deoxyhemoglobin
B. A cold environment
C. Shock compensation
D. Anemia
E. Hypovolemic shock

_____ 59. A yellowish discoloration of the skin, often an indication of liver disease, is known as
A. cyanosis.
B. jaundice.
C. eccyhmosis.
D. erythema.
E. pallor.

_____ 60. Which of the following is a characteristic of toenails related to advanced age?
A. Hard
B. Thick
C. Brittle
D. Yellowish
E. All of the above

_____ 61. Your patient fell from the back of bleacher seats about 15 feet onto pavement below. He has a bluish-purple discoloration around both of his eyes that makes you suspect basilar skull fracture. The finding is called
A. raccoon eyes.
B. Battle's sign.
C. periorbital ecchymosis.
D. retroauricular ecchymosis.
E. either A or C.

_____ 62. When both pupils constrict even though a penlight is shined into only one eye, this is called a(n)
A. consensual response.
B. direct response.
C. simultaneous response.
D. ipsilateral response.
E. none of the above.

_____ 63. A term that describes pupils that are not equal in size is
A. hyphema.
B. anisocoria.
C. glaucoma.
D. hypopyon.
E. none of the above.

_____ 64. In addition to the sense of hearing, which of the following describes a function of the ear?
A. Equalization of pressure during yawning
B. Vibration sensation
C. Balance and head position sense
D. Equalization of body and outside pressure
E. All of the above except B

_____ 65. A medical term for bleeding from the nose is
     A. epistaxis.   D. rhinitis.
     B. otorrhea.   E. none of the above.
     C. rhinorrhea.

_____ 66. The uppermost landmark of the anterior neck is the prominent structure called the
     A. cricoid cartilage.   D. thyroid gland.
     B. thyroid cartilage.   E. jugular vein.
     C. tracheal ring.

_____ 67. The smooth lining that is adherent to the inner wall of the thorax to allow the lungs to glide along the thoracic wall with breathing is the
     A. visceral pleura.   D. pulmonary pleura.
     B. parietal pleura.   E. perineum.
     C. pertioneum.

_____ 68. Where would you be most likely to see retractions associated with forced inspiration caused by partial airway obstruction?
     A. Suprasternal notch   D. All of the above
     B. Intercostal spaces   E. None of the above
     C. Supraclavicular space

_____ 69. Upon percussing a patient's chest, you notice an area of dullness. You should suspect which of the following conditions?
     A. Pneumothorax   D. Pericardial tamponade
     B. Tension pneumothorax   E. Friction rubs
     C. Hemothorax

_____ 70. Fine fizzing or popping sounds in the lungs, reminiscent of the bubbling of a carbonated beverage, are called
     A. rhonchi.   D. wheezes.
     B. stridor.   E. none of the above.
     C. crackles.

_____ 71. When you hear the "lub" of the "lub-dub" cycle of heart sounds, which of the following events is occurring in the heart?
     A. Ejection of blood from the ventricles
     B. Ventricular contraction
     C. Ventricular filling
     D. Closing of the aortic and pulmonic valves
     E. Closing of the tricuspid and mitral valves

_____ 72. A change in which of the following would NOT affect cardiac output?
     A. Heart rate   D. Hematocrit
     B. Cardiac preload   E. Peripheral vascular resistance
     C. Contractile force

_____ 73. All of the following conditions could inhibit the return of venous blood to the heart EXCEPT
     A. peripheral vascular resistance.   D. cardiac tamponade.
     B. hypovolemia.   E. congestive heart failure.
     C. tension pneumothorax.

_____ 74. A bluish discoloration around a patient's umbilicus is termed
     A. Grey Turner's sign.   D. Cullen's sign.
     B. borborygmi.   E. none of the above.
     C. Hering-Breuer's sign.

©2013 Pearson Education, Inc.
Paramedic Care: Principles & Practice, Vol. 3, 4th Ed.

_____ 75. Which of the following is characteristic of hearing high-pitched gurgles and clicks every 5 to 15 seconds while auscultating bowel sounds?
A. Borborygmi
B. Increased bowel motility
C. Absent bowel sounds
D. Normal bowel sounds
E. Ascites

_____ 76. A grating or crunching sound that may be heard as diseased or injured bone surfaces rub together is called
A. palpable fremitus.
B. crepitus.
C. a bruit.
D. a friction rub.
E. subcutaneous emphysema.

_____ 77. Which movement is permitted by the distal and middle joints of the fingers?
A. Abduction/adduction
B. Rotation
C. Flexion/extension
D. Supination/pronation
E. Both C and D

_____ 78. The _____ joint has the greatest range of motion of any joint in the body.
A. shoulder
B. wrist
C. hip
D. elbow
E. ankle

_____ 79. The large muscle that makes up the calf of the leg is called the
A. bicep.
B. tricep.
C. gastrocnemius.
D. hamstring.
E. gracilis anterior.

_____ 80. Which bone is NOT part of the knee joint?
A. Femur
B. Patella
C. Tibia
D. Fibula
E. All of the above

_____ 81. The knee joint is normally allowed what type of motion?
A. Flexion/extension
B. Adduction/abduction
C. Inversion/eversion
D. Limited rotation
E. Both A and D

_____ 82. The region of the spine with the greatest mobility is the _____ region.
A. cervical
B. thoracic
C. lumbar
D. sacral
E. coccygeal

_____ 83. Upon palpating a patient's vertebral process and surrounding muscles, he complains of tenderness. You should suspect that the most likely problem is:
A. a vertebral process fracture.
B. a ligamentous injury.
C. a paravertebral muscular spasm.
D. a herniated intervertebral disk.
E. none of the above.

_____ 84. All of the following findings should make you suspect an occlusion of the proximal artery EXCEPT
A. thrills.
B. pulse deficit.
C. cold limb.
D. poor color in the fingertips.
E. slow capillary refill.

_____ 85. When you find pitting edema, the depression you left in the tissue should resolve within _____ seconds.
A. 2
B. 4
C. 6
D. 8
E. 10

_____ 86. When you document that you performed a complete neurological exam, this means you examined which of the following?
   A. Cranial nerves
   B. Motor system
   C. Reflexes
   D. Sensory system
   E. All of the above

_____ 87. Which is a characteristic of normal speech?
   A. Inflected
   B. Clear and strong
   C. Fluent and articulate
   D. Variable in volume
   E. All of the above

_____ 88. You have documented that a patient suffers from aphasia. This means the patient has which of the following problems?
   A. Defective speech caused by motor deficits
   B. Voice changes due to vocal cord problems
   C. Defective language due to a neurologic problem
   D. Voice changes due to aging
   E. None of the above

_____ 89. Memories are categorized as any of the following EXCEPT
   A. intermediate.
   B. verifiable.
   C. redux.
   D. remote.
   E. retrograde.

_____ 90. To test a patient's extraoccular eye movements, which figure should you trace with your finger before the patient's eyes?
   A. An "X"
   B. An "H"
   C. A "1"
   D. A large "O"
   E. Any of the above

_____ 91. Which of the following functions is mediated by the pyramidal pathway of the spinal cord?
   A. Voluntary muscle control
   B. Involuntary muscle control
   C. Dermatome sensation
   D. Visceral sensation
   E. Vasoconstriction

_____ 92. Which would you expect to see in a patient who has damage to the extrapyramidal pathways?
   A. Abnormal posture
   B. Abnormal gait
   C. Involuntary movement
   D. Increased muscle tone
   E. All of the above

_____ 93. The section of skin that is provided with sensation by a specific pair of spinal nerves is referred to as a(n)
   A. afferent region.
   B. sensory topographic region.
   C. myotome.
   D. dermatome.
   E. both A and C.

_____ 94. A patient has a positive Babinski reflex if which of the following occurs when you stroke the bottom of the foot?
   A. The big toe plantar flexes while other toes dorsiflex.
   B. The big toe plantar flexes while other toes fan out.
   C. The big toe dorsiflexes while other toes fan out.
   D. The big toe dorsiflexes while other toes plantar flex.
   E. All toes plantar flex.

_____ 95. A child should first recognize his parents' faces when he is _____ old.
   A. 2 months
   B. 6 months
   C. 8 months
   D. 10 months
   E. 1 year

©2013 Pearson Education, Inc.
Paramedic Care: Principles & Practice, Vol. 3, 4th Ed.

_____ 96. By what age does an infant begin to sit by himself?
- **A.** 2 to 4 months
- **B.** 4 to 6 months
- **C.** 6 to 8 months
- **D.** 10 months to 1 year
- **E.** 1 year or later

Chapter 6: Patient Monitoring Technology

_____ 97. The usual lead for obtaining a cardiac rhythm strip is lead
- **A.** aVR.
- **B.** aVF.
- **C.** I.
- **D.** II.
- **E.** III.

_____ 98. Each 1-mm square on a standard ECG represents a time period of _____ second.
- **A.** .02
- **B.** .04
- **C.** .06
- **D.** .12
- **E.** .20

_____ 99. The first positive deflection in a normal lead II ECG rhythm strip is the _____ wave.
- **A.** Q
- **B.** R
- **C.** S
- **D.** P
- **E.** T

_____ 100. An ST segment myocardial infarction is diagnosed if the ST segment is elevated in lead II.
- **A.** True
- **B.** False

_____ 101. Which of the following is a DISADVANTAGE of a standard 12-lead ECG?
- **A.** It cannot show conduction defects in the His-Purkinje system.
- **B.** It only shows positive deflections.
- **C.** It cannot show most problems with the left side of the heart.
- **D.** You cannot assess the ST segment.
- **E.** It cannot show most problems with the right ventricle and posterior left ventricle.

_____ 102. What is the most important reason that paramedics obtain a 12-lead ECG in the prehospital setting?
- **A.** Unknown—still being studied
- **B.** To rule out acute coronary syndrome
- **C.** To monitor the cardiac rhythm
- **D.** To identify patients with congestive heart failure
- **E.** To shorten the time for STEMI patients to receive reperfusion therapy

_____ 103. The Bohr effect describes the tendency for hemoglobin to more readily release oxygen molecules in conditions of low pH.
- **A.** True
- **B.** False

_____ 104. You should consider administering supplemental oxygen when a patient's SpO_2 drops below _____ percent.
- **A.** 100
- **B.** 98
- **C.** 95
- **D.** 92
- **E.** 90

_____ **105.** When analyzing $ETCO_2$, which of the following would be an acceptable value?
  A. 29 mmHg
  B. 33 mmHg
  C. 38 mmHg
  D. 41 mmHg
  E. Both C and D

_____ **106.** Waveform capnometry is more reliable than continuous colorimetric capnography.
  A. True
  B. False

_____ **107.** Waveform capnography can be used to determine the effectiveness of chest compressions in a patient in whom cardiopulmonary resuscitation (CPR) is being performed.
  A. True
  B. False

_____ **108.** For which of the following situations would monitoring of methemoglobin be most useful?
  A. To assess for return of spontaneous circulation in cardiac arrest
  B. For patients receiving intravenous nitrates
  C. To continuously monitor endotracheal tube placement
  D. For patients with acute asthma
  E. For patients receiving prolonged 100 percent oxygen

_____ **109.** Hyperglycemia is a condition in which the blood glucose level is above _____ mg/dL.
  A. 80
  B. 100
  C. 120
  D. 140
  E. 160

_____ **110.** In which type of patient is it important to determine a blood glucose level?
  A. Known diabetics
  B. Patients with altered mental status
  C. Alcoholics
  D. Patients with hepatitis
  E. All of the above

_____ **111.** The order in which blood tubes are filled when obtaining venous blood samples is not important.
  A. True
  B. False

_____ **112.** Abdominal ultrasound in trauma is only reliable when there are large amounts of blood within the abdominal cavity.
  A. True
  B. False

Chapter 7: Patient Assessment in the Field

_____ **113.** Which step in patient assessment is always performed during transport to the hospital, even when patients seem stable?
  A. Scene size-up
  B. Primary assessment
  C. Focused history and physical exam
  D. Detailed physical exam
  E. Reassessment

©2013 Pearson Education, Inc.
Paramedic Care: Principles & Practice, Vol. 3, 4th Ed.

_____114. All of the following are involved in the scene size-up EXCEPT
    A. consideration of c-spine.
    B. general impression of the patient.
    C. location of all patients.
    D. analysis of mechanism of injury/nature of the illness.
    E. scene safety.

_____115. When you approach a patient and see that he does not appear to be conscious or breathing normally, your next steps are represented by the mnemonic
    A. ABC.
    B. OPQRST-ASPN.
    C. CAB.
    D. SAMPLE.
    E. AEIOU-TIPS.

_____116. Which assessment component is performed first for all patients, regardless of the nature of the call?
    A. Primary assessment
    B. Initial assessment
    C. Secondary assessment
    D. Scene size-up
    E. Focused history and physical exam

_____117. Which of the following is NOT a patient classification for the purposes of determining how to approach the secondary assessment?
    A. Responsive medical patient
    B. Unresponsive medical patient
    C. Pediatric patient with altered consciousness
    D. Minor trauma patient
    E. Major trauma patient

_____118. Which of the following is used as a criterion in the initial determination of whether a patient should be transported to a trauma center?
    A. Gender
    B. Serious clinical findings
    C. Pulse oximetry reading
    D. Blood glucose level
    E. Waveform capnography

_____119. When a patient has subcutaneous emphysema, this means that you have noted which of the following in the physical exam?
    A. A grating sensation
    B. Air trapped under the skin
    C. Air leaking from the respiratory system
    D. Retraction of the tissues between the ribs
    E. Fluid accumulation just beneath the skin

_____120. Which of the following should you suspect if you note intercostal or suprasternal retractions during your physical examination?
    A. Tension pneumothorax
    B. Subcutaneous emphysema
    C. Airway obstruction or restriction
    D. Flail chest
    E. Either B or D

_____121. While assessing a patient's injured arm, you find that his motor function is present, but distal to the elbow the limb is cool and pale and you cannot palpate pulses in the wrist. Which of the following should be highest on your list of differential diagnoses?
    A. Neurologic compromise
    B. Vascular compromise
    C. Both a vascular and a neurologic compromise
    D. Spinal injury
    E. Peripheral nerve root injury

_____ 122. Even as you are completing the history of a patient who is complaining of chest pain, which of the following will you direct your team to do?
  A. Attach a cardiac monitor
  B. Administer oxygen
  C. Take vital signs
  D. Start an IV, if appropriate
  E. All of the above

_____ 123. The concern that caused a patient to request your help is the patient's
  A. presenting problem.
  B. differential diagnosis.
  C. field diagnosis.
  D. chief complaint.
  E. present illness.

_____ 124. You should suspect impaired venous return if a patient's jugular veins remain full when he is sitting at _____ or higher.
  A. 15°
  B. 30°
  C. 45°
  D. 60°
  E. 90°

_____ 125. Hyperresonance in response to percussion of the chest is an indication of which of the following problems?
  A. Pleural effusion
  B. Pulmonary edema
  C. Pneumonia
  D. Emphysema
  E. None of the above

_____ 126. If you are checking a patient's abdomen for an abnormal pulsation of the aorta, you should palpate
  A. just right of the umbilicus.
  B. just left of the umbilicus.
  C. along a line from the umbilicus to the middle symphysis pubis.
  D. just beneath the xiphoid process.
  E. anywhere in the abdomen.

_____ 127. Which problem causes an accumulation of fluid in the abdomen?
  A. Hypovolemia
  B. Aortic aneurysm
  C. Emphysema
  D. Gastric ulcer disease
  E. Cirrhosis of the liver

_____ 128. When a patient's pupils are not the same size, you should record the finding as
  A. Cullen's sign.
  B. anisocoria.
  C. consensual response.
  D. accommodation.
  E. Bell's palsy.

_____ 129. For which classification of patient is a detailed, head-to-toe exam most important?
  A. The severe trauma patient
  B. The minor trauma patient
  C. The responsive medical patient
  D. The unresponsive medical patient
  E. Both A and D

_____ 130. Which of the following can only be done if you continue to reassess your patient during transport?
  A. Identifying trends in the patient's condition
  B. Revising the field diagnosis
  C. Making changes in the management plan
  D. Documenting the effects of interventions
  E. All of the above

©2013 Pearson Education, Inc.
Paramedic Care: Principles & Practice, Vol. 3, 4th Ed.

SPECIAL PROJECTS

Locating Auscultation Points

On the following illustration, identify where you would locate the stethoscope disk or bell to auscultate breath and heart (pulmonic, aortic, mitral, and tricuspid areas and PMI) sounds.

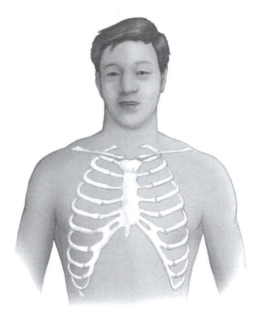

See the crossword puzzle on the next page.

Crossword Puzzle

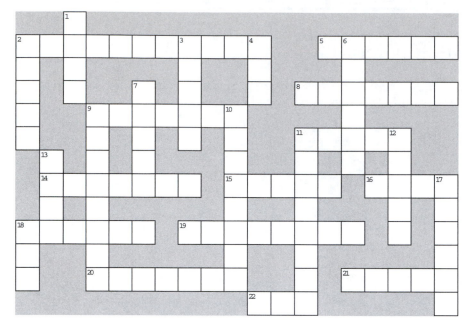

Across

2. Rapid heartbeat

5. Wound

8. High-pitched respiratory sounds

9. Related to the heart

11. _____ complaint: the reason the patient called EMS

14. Fluid build-up in the abdomen

15. Written defamation of another person

16. Type of respirator used when treating a suspected tuberculosis patient

18. Involuntary response to a stimulus

19. Acute alteration in mental function

20. Loud, high-pitched inspiratory wheeze

21. Elements of the head assessment (abbr.)

22. Advanced life support (abbr.)

Down

1. Repeat a verbal order

2. _____ volume: normal respiratory volume

3. Basic EMS communication device

4. Against medical advice (abbr.)

6. Vomitus

7. Sound indicating turbulent blood flow

9. Light, popping, nonmusical inspiratory sounds

10. Type of phone service used by many EMS systems

11. Grating sensation or sound

12. _____ diagnosis: prehospital evaluation of the patient's condition and its causes

13. Questionnaire used for suspected alcoholic patients

17. Severity of an injury or illness

18. Review of the systems (abbr.)

WORKBOOK ANSWER KEY

Note: Throughout the Answer Key, textbook page references are shown in italics.

Chapter 1: Scene Size-Up

Content Self-Evaluation

MULTIPLE CHOICE

1.	E	*p. 2*	7.	E	*p. 6*	13.	D	*p. 14*
2.	B	*p. 4*	8.	C	*p. 6*	14.	E	*p. 15*
3.	A	*p. 5*	9.	A	*p. 10*	15.	C	*p. 15*
4.	C	*p. 5*	10.	D	*p. 13*	16.	E	*p. 16*
5.	A	*p. 5*	11.	B	*p. 12*			
6.	E	*p. 6*	12.	A	*p. 14*			

MATCHING

p. 5

17. B
18. E
19. D
20. A
21. E
22. C

SHORT ANSWER

p. 8

23. A) Contains or has the potential to contain a hazardous atmosphere, B) Contains material that has the potential to engulf an entrant, C) Has walls that converge inward or floors that slope downward and taper into a smaller area that could trap or asphyxiate an entrant, D) Contains any other recognized safety or health hazard, such as unguarded machinery, exposed live wires, or heat stress.

p. 9

24. A) Liquids, gases, solids, corrosives, poisons, nerve agents, and toxic industrial materials, B) Viruses, bacteria, biotoxins, C) Nuclear weapons, dirty bombs, nuclear waste, D) Gunpowder, TNT, dynamite, improvised explosive devices.

p. 9

25. A) Don't rush in, B) Don't assume anything, C) Don't become a victim, D) Don't test a foreign substance.

Special Project: Scene Size-Up Exercise

A. Traffic, unstable vehicle, spilled gasoline/fire, stream contamination, unstable/slippery surfaces, hazardous chemicals, broken glass/jagged metal, hot surfaces.
B. Structural collapse, debris, confined space, electrical hazards, explosion, body substances.
C. Fast water, drowning, hypothermia.

CHAPTER 2: Primary Assessment

Content Self-Evaluation

MULTIPLE CHOICE

1.	C	*p. 21*	8.	B	*p. 25*	15.	C	*p. 25*
2.	A	*p. 21*	9.	D	*p. 25*	16.	B	*p. 26*
3.	E	*p. 22*	10.	A	*p. 25*	17.	C	*p. 25*
4.	C	*p. 22*	11.	C	*p. 28*	18.	A	*p. 27*
5.	A	*p. 23*	12.	B	*p. 26*	19.	A	*p. 28*
6.	C	*p. 23*	13.	E	*p. 26*	20.	B	*p. 21*
7.	B	*p. 23*	14.	C	*p. 24*			

LISTING

p. 21

21. Forming a general impression.
22. Stabilizing the cervical spine, if needed.
23. Assessing a baseline mental status.
24. Assessing and managing the airway.
25. Assessing and managing breathing.
26. Assessing and managing circulation.
27. Determining priorities of care and transport.

SPECIAL PROJECT: Assessing the Mental Status

Review pp. 23–24.

A. An alert patient is awake as evidenced by open eyes, but may either be oriented or confused.
V. A patient who is responsive to verbal stimuli may appear to be sleeping but verbalizes, opens his eyes, or makes some movement in response to your voice.
P. A patient who does not respond to voice is responsive to pain if he opens his eyes, makes a noise, or moves in response to a painful stimulus.
U. An unresponsive patient does not give any kind of response to verbal or painful stimuli.

CHAPTER 3: Therapeutic Communications

MULTIPLE CHOICE

1.	C	*p. 40*
2.	C	*p. 40*
3.	B	*p. 38*
4.	B	*p. 40*
5.	B	*p. 41*
6.	A	*p. 47*
7.	A	*p. 48*
8.	E	*pp. 43–44*

MATCHING

p. 41

9. C
10. D
11. E
12. A
13. B

CHAPTER 4: History Taking

Content Self-Evaluation

MULTIPLE CHOICE

1.	D	p. 53	8.	B	p. 54	15.	C	p. 56
2.	B	p. 53	9.	C	p. 55	16.	D	p. 57
3.	B	p. 54	10.	B	p. 54	17.	E	p. 59
4.	C	p. 53	11.	A	p. 54	18.	A	p. 60
5.	A	p. 54	12.	B	p. 55	19.	E	p. 60
6.	C	p. 55	13.	C	p. 56			
7.	B	p. 54	14.	E	p. 56			

MATCHING

pp. 55–60

20.	E	24.	A	28.	Q	32.	T
21.	C	25.	S	29.	P	33.	Q
22.	D	26.	P	30	O	34.	O
23.	B	27.	R	31.	R		

SHORT ANSWER

pp. 60–61

35. The differential field diagnosis is a listing of the primary problems that could cause the chief complaint. The final field diagnosis is the most likely primary problem responsible for the patient's chief complaint, history, signs, and symptoms, based upon the patient assessment.

SPECIAL PROJECT: History of the Present Illness

O. (onset of the problem): rapid onset while jogging.

P. (provacative/palliative factors): mild pain while deep breathing.

Q. (quality of pain): sharp, stabbing.

R. (radiation/region of pain): most left of sternum at 3rd intercostal space, with no radiation.

S. (severity): 8 on a scale of 1 to 10.

T. (time of onset): sudden, with no preceding events.

AS. (associated symptoms): none reported.

PN. (pertinent negatives): denies COPD, asthma, and history of heart problems.

CHAPTER 5: Secondary Assessment

Content Self-Evaluation

MULTIPLE CHOICE

1.	A	p. 67	18.	E	p. 79	35.	B	p. 84
2.	B	p. 69	19.	B	p. 79	36.	D	p. 87
3.	A	p. 68	20.	C	p. 79	37.	E	p. 87
4.	C	p. 67	21.	D	p. 79	38.	E	p. 90
5.	B	p. 68	22.	C	p. 82	39.	C	p. 91
6.	C	p. 68	23.	D	p. 70	40.	D	p. 91
7.	A	p. 68	24.	D	p. 70	41.	A	p. 94
8.	A	p. 69	25.	B	p. 70	42.	B	p. 94
9.	C	p. 79	26.	B	p. 80	43.	C	p. 96
10.	B	p. 78	27.	D	p. 78	44.	E	p. 96
11.	C	p. 78	28.	B	p. 79	45.	A	p. 101
12.	A	p. 78	29.	A	p. 76	46.	B	p. 103
13.	E	p. 76	30.	E	p. 81	47.	B	p. 106
14.	A	p. 76	31.	C	p. 81	48.	B	p. 106
15.	D	p. 76	32.	B	p. 81	49.	B	p. 106
16.	C	p. 79	33.	E	p. 81	50.	E	p. 107
17.	A	p. 79	34.	A	p. 83	51.	B	p. 107

52.	A	p. 107	70.	C	p. 136	88.	B	p. 93
53.	C	p. 107	71.	D	p. 136	89.	A	p. 94
54.	C	p. 107	72.	E	p. 137	90.	C	p. 147
55.	A	p. 109	73.	A	p. 142	91.	D	p. 149
56.	D	p. 116	74.	E	p. 143	92.	A	p. 149
57.	A	p. 114	75.	B	p. 144	93.	E	p. 149
58.	E	p. 114	76.	D	p. 144	94.	D	p. 150
59.	D	p. 111	77.	C	p. 118	95.	E	p. 150
60.	A	p. 111	78.	A	p. 118	96.	A	p. 150
61.	C	p. 119	79.	D	p. 118	97.	B	p. 152
62.	D	p. 121	80.	E	p. 118	98.	D	p. 153
63.	D	p. 112	81.	E	p. 146	99.	C	p. 152
64.	A	p. 124	82.	E	p. 71	100.	C	p. 155
65.	B	p. 128	83.	E	p. 72	101.	E	p. 71
66.	C	p. 128	84.	B	p. 76	102.	A	p. 72
67.	B	p. 129	85.	C	p. 76	103.	B	p. 72
68.	C	p. 131	86.	D	p. 74	104.	B	p. 72
69.	A	p. 132	87.	D	p. 74	105.	C	p. 72

MATCHING

pp. 147

106.	L, M	110.	G, X	114.	F, T
107.	B, P	111.	D, U	115.	I, N
108.	H, W	112.	K, Q	116.	E, O
109.	C, S	113.	A, V	117.	J, R

SPECIAL PROJECT: Vital Signs

Pulse: (p. 78) Normal adult pulse rates are between 60 and 100 beats per minute. The pulse is normally regular and strong.

Respirations: (p. 76) Normal adult respiratory rate is between 12 and 18 breaths per minute, effortless, and regular. The normal adult tidal volume is about 500 mL.

Blood pressure: (p. 79) Normal adult blood pressure is approximately 120/80, but the systolic pressure ranges from 100 to 135 mmHg and the diastolic pressure ranges from 60 to 80 mmHg. Normal pulse pressure is 30 to 40 mmHg.

Temperature: (p. 82) Normal body temperature is approximately 98.6 degrees Fahrenheit or 37 degrees Celsius.

SPECIAL PROJECT: Range of Motion Exercise

Upper Extremity

Joint	Flexion/ Extension	Rotation	Other Motion
Wrist	90/70		(Medial/lateral) 20/45
Elbow	160/0		(Supination/pronation) 90/90
Shoulder	180/50	(Internal/external) 90/90	(Abduction/adduction) 180/75

Lower Extremity

Joint	Flexion/ Extension	Rotation	Other Motion
Ankle	Dorsiflex/ plantar flex 20/45		(Inversion/eversion) 30/20
Knee	135/90		
Hip	120/0	(External/internal) 40/45	(Abduction) 90

©2013 Pearson Education, Inc.
Paramedic Care: Principles & Practice, Vol. 3, 4th Ed.

CHAPTER 6: Patient Monitoring Technology

Content Self-Evaluation

MULTIPLE CHOICE

1.	A	*p. 165*	11.	B	*p. 180*	21.	B	*p. 190*
2.	D	*p. 167*	12.	A	*p. 181*	22.	A	*p. 192*
3.	B	*p. 167*	13.	C	*p. 181*	23.	C	*p. 193*
4.	B	*p. 168*	14.	C	*p. 183*	24.	D	*p. 194*
5.	D	*p. 168*	15.	D	*p. 183*	25.	E	*p. 194*
6.	B	*p. 170*	16.	E	*p. 183*	26.	B	*p. 196*
7.	C	*p. 173*	17.	B	*p. 184*	27.	D	*p. 198*
8.	A	*p. 175*	18.	A	*p. 185*	28.	A	*p. 200*
9.	E	*p. 175*	19.	A	*p. 187*	29.	B	*p. 202*
10.	E	*p. 178*	20.	E	*p. 187*	30.	A	*p. 202*

MATCHING

p. 178

31.	C	36.	E	41.	G
32.	C	37.	E	42.	F
33.	D	38.	A	43.	B
34.	D	39.	A		
35.	D	40.	G		

SPECIAL PROJECT: Deciding When to Use Patient Monitoring Technology

Continuous ECG monitoring (*p. 171*)**:** ECG monitoring is a part of any patient receiving advanced life support procedures, and is particularly important for patients with chest pain or abnormalities in pulse rate or rhythm.

12-lead ECG (*p. 178*)**:** The 12-lead ECG is important in the early recognition and treatment of ST segment elevation myocardial infarction.

Pulse oximetry (*p. 182*)**:** Pulse oximetry is used when there is any suspicion that a patient is at risk for hypoxia.

Capnography (*p. 185*)**:** Capnography, particularly waveform capnography, is important in many instances. Two important reasons for using capnography are (1) ro confirm and monitor placement of endotracheal tubes, and (2) to assist in determining return of spontaneous circulation in cardiac arrest.

Glucometry (*p. 194*)**:** Glucometry must be used in any patient with an altered mental status and in diabetic patients. It also can be useful in assessing patients with other conditions that increase the risk of hypoglycemia.

CHAPTER 7: Patient Assessment in the Field

Content Self-Evaluation

MULTIPLE CHOICE

1.	A	*p. 207*	11.	B	*p. 212*	21.	C	*p. 220*
2.	E	*p. 223*	12.	C	*p. 212*	22.	A	*p. 220*
3.	C	*p. 207*	13.	B	*p. 212*	23.	D	*p. 220*
4.	A	*p. 207*	14.	D	*p. 215*	24.	B	*p. 220*
5.	B	*p. 208*	15.	B	*p. 215*	25.	E	*p. 220*
6.	C	*p. 209*	16.	D	*p. 216*	26.	B	*p. 221*
7.	D	*p. 209*	17.	C	*p. 216*	27.	E	*p. 207*
8.	B	*p. 210*	18.	E	*p. 218*	28.	E	*p. 225*
9.	E	*p. 210*	19.	D	*p. 219*			
10.	A	*p. 211*	20.	B	*p. 219*			

MATCHING

p. 226

29.	B	33.	C	37.	A
30.	D	34.	B	38.	D
31.	A	35.	A	39.	E
32.	A	36.	C		

SPECIAL PROJECT: Summarizing the Clinical Reasoning Process

pp. 226-227

Form a concept: Gather observations from assessing the scene, asking questions, and examining the patient.

Interpret the data: Compare your observations to your knowledge and experience to determine the most likely cause of the patient's problem.

Apply the principles: Develop a treatment plan and make decisions about management.

Evaluate the results: Reassess the patient and the effects of your interventions.

Reflect on the case: Make every case a learning experience by obtaining feedback on your decision-making process.

Patient Assessment: Content Review

Content Self-Evaluation

CHAPTER 1: SCENE SIZE-UP

1.	E	*p. 2*	5.	D	*p. 13*
2.	B	*p. 5*	6.	A	*p. 12*
3.	C	*p. 5*	7.	E	*p. 14*
4.	E	*p. 6*	8.	E	*p. 16*

CHAPTER 2: PRIMARY ASSESSMENT

9.	C	*p. 21*	13.	D	*p. 25*	17.	B	*p. 24*
10.	A	*p. 22*	14.	B	*p. 25*	18.	C	*p. 25*
11.	E	*p. 23*	15.	A	*p. 25*	19.	A	*p. 28*
12.	C	*p. 23*	16.	C	*p. 28*	20.	B	*p. 21*

CHAPTER 3: THERAPEUTIC COMMUNICATIONS

21.	A	*p. 40*	24.	B	*p. 40*	27.	B	*p. 48*
22.	D	*p. 40*	25.	B	*p. 41*			
23.	B	*p. 38*	26.	A	*p. 47*			

CHAPTER 4: HISTORY TAKING

28.	D	*p. 53*	32.	B	*p. 54*	36.	A	*p. 60*
29.	C	*p. 53*	33.	A	*p. 54*	37.	E	*p. 60*
30.	B	*p. 54*	34.	E	*p. 56*			
31.	E	*p. 55*	35.	D	*p. 57*			

CHAPTER 5: SECONDARY ASSESSMENT

38.	A	*p. 67*	49.	B	*p. 79*	60.	E	*p. 87*
39.	B	*p. 69*	50.	D	*p. 79*	61.	E	*p. 90*
40.	A	*p. 68*	51.	C	*p. 82*	62.	A	*p. 94*
41.	A	*p. 68*	52.	D	*p. 70*	63.	B	*p. 94*
42.	B	*p. 69*	53.	B	*p. 70*	64.	C	*p. 96*
43.	B	*p. 78*	54.	D	*p. 80*	65.	A	*p. 101*
44.	C	*p. 78*	55.	B	*p. 79*	66.	B	*p. 103*
45.	E	*p. 76*	56.	E	*p. 81*	67.	B	*p. 106*
46.	D	*p. 76*	57.	C	*p. 81*	68.	D	*p. 106*
47.	C	*p. 79*	58.	A	*p. 83*	69.	C	*p. 107*
48.	E	*p. 79*	59.	B	*p. 84*	70.	C	*p. 107*

71.	E	*p. 114*	80.	D	*p. 136*	89.	A	*p. 74*
72.	D	*p. 111*	81.	E	*p. 137*	90.	B	*p. 93*
73.	B	*p. 111*	82.	A	*p. 142*	91.	A	*p. 149*
74.	D	*p. 121*	83.	D	*p. 144*	92.	E	*p. 149*
75.	D	*p. 112*	84.	A	*p. 118*	93.	D	*p. 153*
76.	B	*p. 128*	85.	E	*p. 118*	94.	C	*p. 152*
77.	C	*p. 128*	86.	E	*p. 146*	95.	A	*p. 72*
78.	A	*p. 132*	87.	E	*p. 72*	96.	B	*p. 72*
79.	C	*p. 136*	88.	C	*p. 76*			

CHAPTER 6: PATIENT MONITORING TECHNOLOGY

97.	D	*p. 167*	103.	B	*p. 181*	109.	D	*p. 194*
98.	B	*p. 168*	104.	C	*p. 183*	110.	E	*p. 194*
99.	D	*p. 170*	105.	E	*p. 184*	111.	B	*p. 196*
100.	B	*p. 175*	106.	A	*p. 185*	112.	B	*p. 202*
101.	E	*p. 178*	107.	A	*p. 190*			
102.	E	*p. 181*	108.	B	*p. 194*			

CHAPTER 7: PATIENT ASSESSMENT IN THE FIELD

113.	A	*p. 223*	119.	B	*p. 212*	125.	D	*p. 220*
114.	B	*p. 207*	120.	C	*p. 212*	126.	B	*p. 220*
115.	C	*p. 207*	121.	B	*p. 215*	127.	E	*p. 220*
116.	D	*p. 207*	122.	E	*p. 218*	128.	B	*p. 221*
117.	C	*p. 209*	123.	D	*p. 219*	129.	E	*p. 207*
118.	B	*p. 210*	124.	C	*p. 220*	130.	E	*p. 225*

SPECIAL PROJECT: Locating Auscultation Points

See pp. 108 and 114.

Lung sounds: every 5 cm along the midclavicular lines

PMI: 5th intercostal space, left midclavicular line

S1: lower left sternal border

S2: 2nd intercostal space, near sternum

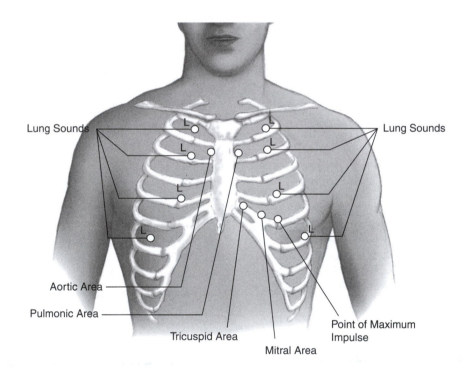

©2013 Pearson Education, Inc.
Paramedic Care: Principles & Practice, Vol. 3, 4th Ed.

			E													
T	A	C	H	Y	C	A	R	D	I	A		L	E	S	I	O	N
I		H				A		M			M				
D		O		B		D		A		W	H	E	E	Z	E	S
A		C	A	R	D	I	A	C			S			
L		R	U	O		E		C	H	I	E	F	
	C	A	I		L		R	S	I	
A	S	C	I	T	E	S	L	I	B	E	L	H	E	P	A
G	K		U		P		L	C
R	E	F	L	E	X	D	E	L	I	R	I	U	M	D	U
O	E		A		T		I
S	S	T	R	I	D	O	R	U	H	E	E	N	T
A	L	S	Y

©2013 Pearson Education, Inc.
Paramedic Care: Principles & Practice, Vol. 3, 4th Ed.

PATIENT SCENARIO FLASH CARDS

In order to help you learn the process of investigating the chief complaint and obtaining the past medical history, this Workbook includes a series of flash cards. Each one contains the dispatch and scene size-up information and then asks you to question either the patient's chief complaint or the past medical history.

Using the flash cards is a two-person exercise. Work with another member of your class, a paramedic or an EMT from your service, or someone else knowledgeable in emergency medical care. Cut the cards and shuffle them. Have your partner choose a card at random and read the dispatch and scene size-up information aloud to you. He should read the patient information to himself and prepare to play the role of the patient. You should then try to determine the patient history by questioning him using the elements of the SAMPLE mnemonic. Your partner should then choose other cards, and the two of you should repeat the exercise until you feel comfortable in gathering the patient history.

Then have your partner repeat the exercise, reading the dispatch and scene size-up information and role-playing the part of the patient with symptoms associated with the chief complaint. You should then question him about the chief complaint using the OPQRST-ASPN mnemonic. When you feel comfortable with the process of questioning for the chief complaint, repeat the exercise with your partner, using information on both sides of the card. When you have gathered all the information you can, create a patient report like the one you would provide when arriving at the emergency department with your patient. Also attempt to determine the field diagnosis for the patient (listed at the bottom of the chief complaint card). Repeat the exercise until you are comfortable with the entire process.

PATIENT HISTORY

The patient history examines critical elements of the patient's past medical history, including the elements of the SAMPLE history mnemonic. (The "S," for signs and symptoms, is investigated during the questioning about the chief complaint.)

A—allergies	Ask about any allergies or adverse reactions to drugs, foods, and so on.
M—medications	Ask about any prescribed medications, then over-the-counter ones.
P—past medical history	Ask about recent surgeries, hospitalizations, and physician care.
L—last oral intake	Ask about the most recent meal and any fluids ingested.
E—events before the incident	Ask about activities and symptoms preceding the incident.

CHIEF COMPLAINT

During the investigation of the chief complaint, question the patient about the major symptoms of the problem to help form a field diagnosis. Investigate your patient's complaints by using the OPQRST-ASPN mnemonic.

O (onset)	Ask about how the symptoms developed and what the patient was doing at the time.
P (palliation/provocation)	Ask about what makes the symptoms better or worse.
Q (quality)	Ask the patient to describe the nature of the pain or discomfort.
R (region/radiation)	Ask where the symptom and related symptoms are found.
S (severity)	Ask the patient to rate the pain on a scale from 1 to 10 (worst pain).
T (time)	Ask about when the symptoms first appeared and how they progressed.
AS (associated symptoms)	Ask about other or associated symptoms.
PN (pertinent negatives)	Investigate likely and related signs and symptoms.

During this exercise, do not try to develop standard questions for each element of the investigation. Rather, let your patient's condition, the nature of the problem, and—later in your career—your experience guide your questioning to garner the pertinent medical information.

Card 1 PATIENT HISTORY

Dispatch Information: Responding to a residence for a patient complaining of chest pain

Scene Size-Up: Small but clean home with the patient seated on the couch, in obvious pain, and clutching his chest; no hazards noted.

Medical History

A—anesthetic at the dentist's office ("caine" family)

M—nitroglycerin and calcium supplements

P—sees his doctor yearly but doesn't have any medical problems

L—breakfast an hour ago, two eggs, toast, and coffee

E—watching television, nothing unusual

Card 2 PATIENT HISTORY

Dispatch Information: Responding to a local movie theater for a man with abdominal pain

Scene Size-Up: A crowd surrounds a man seated in the lobby; no hazards noted.

Medical History

A—doesn't know of any

M—none

P—pelvic fracture 3 years ago (auto collision)

L—a large prime rib dinner 2 hours ago with a couple of gin and tonics

E—just sitting in the movie when this pain began and became progressively worse

---

Card 3 PATIENT HISTORY

Dispatch Information: Seizure at the arcade

Scene Size-Up: You are directed to the manager's office, where you find a rather lethargic young female; no hazards are noted.

Medical History

A—doesn't know

M—Dilantin® and phenobarbital, but hasn't been taking them

P—serious auto collision and then seizures

L—had a light lunch an hour ago

E—just felt warm; then blacked out

Card 1 CHIEF COMPLAINT

O—sudden onset, 15 minutes ago

P—nothing, including nitro, makes it better or worse

Q—dull

R—substernal with some right arm numbness

S—12 out of 10, more than ever before

T—while watching TV

AS—some nausea

PN—no dizziness or dyspnea

(Field diagnosis: myocardial infarction)

Card 2 CHIEF COMPLAINT

O—gradual onset; started about 1 hour ago and got worse

P—bending over gives some relief

Q—dull, cramping-like pain

R—right upper quadrant with some pain in the right shoulder

S—10 on a scale of 1 to 10

T—ate a prime rib dinner 2 hours ago, watching a movie

AS—some nausea

PN—none noted

(Field diagnosis: gallbladder inflammation [cholecystitis])

Card 3 CHIEF COMPLAINT

O—just had a warm feeling; then blacked out

P—none

Q—bystander states the patient tensed, arched her back, then seized

R—bystander states seizure began with everything shaking

S—generalized motor seizure

T—watching the lights on an arcade game; then experienced a warm feeling, collapsed, and awoke feeling tired

AS—tongue bitten and bleeding

PN—no headache

(Field diagnosis: epilepsy)

Card 4 PATIENT HISTORY

Dispatch Information: Responding to a nursing home for a resident with problems breathing

Scene Size-Up: You are directed by staff to an elderly patient, in bed on oxygen, and in noticeable distress; no hazards noted.

Medical History

A—shellfish

M—28 percent oxygen via Venturi mask

P—emphysema (30 pack/year smoker) and a weak heart

L—light breakfast 4 hours ago and a glass of milk an hour ago

E—just lying here, knitting

Card 5 PATIENT HISTORY

Dispatch Information: Patient with abdominal pain at the high school

Scene Size-Up: At the high school nurse's office, you find a young female teenager curled up on the couch; no hazards noted.

Medical History

A—none

M—antibiotic for infection

P—none

L—breakfast this morning

E—twinge of pain began earlier this morning and grew worse

Card 6 PATIENT HISTORY

Dispatch Information: Dispatched to the local library for a man who has collapsed

Scene Size-Up: An older, well-dressed gentleman is lying on the floor in a pool of his own urine; no hazards noted.

Medical History

A—none known

M—daily aspirin and digitalis for heart disease

P—cardiac dysrhythmias

L—dinner about an hour ago

E—just sitting and reading when a headache developed

Card 4 CHIEF COMPLAINT

O—slow progression of difficulty breathing

P—any movement or stress makes it worse

Q—general fatigue and a "tight" chest

R—limited to the chest

S—intensity of dyspnea, 8 out of 10

T—progressed slowly, started 2 hours ago

AS—none

PN—no pitting edema or jugular vein distension

(Field diagnosis: exacerbation of COPD)

Card 5 CHIEF COMPLAINT

O—the pain began this morning and has gradually increased

P—somewhat more comfortable in the fetal position

Q—"crampy"

R—localized to the left lower quadrant

S—pain is 9 on a scale of 1 to 10

T—gradually increasing since morning, nothing unusual in diet or activity

AS—last period spotty, not the usual flow

PN—appendix was removed last year

(Field diagnosis: ectopic pregnancy)

Card 6 CHIEF COMPLAINT

O—developed a headache and then just collapsed

P—nothing affects the pain or paralysis

Q—throbbing headache; full, one-sided paralysis

R—left-sided paralysis of both extremities

S—headache pain is 10 on a scale of 1 to 10

T—reading preceded symptoms

AS—incontinence, difficulty speaking and understanding

PN—pupils normal and reactive

(Field diagnosis: CVA—stroke)

Card 7 PATIENT HISTORY

Dispatch Information: Proceed to a local restaurant for an unruly and disoriented person.

Scene Size-Up: Police are already at the scene, where a young woman who looks anxious is seated in a booth; no hazards noted.

Medical History

A—sulfa drugs

M—insulin subcutaneously twice per day

P—juvenile-onset (type I) diabetes

L—ate a small breakfast about 8 hours ago

E—took insulin just after breakfast

Card 8 PATIENT HISTORY

Dispatch Information: Dispatched to high school gym for a "weak student"

Scene Size-Up: A young male is seated on the bleachers in obvious distress; no hazards noted.

Medical History

A—tetanus toxoid

M—none

P—none but had sports physical last month; everything was OK

L—a good-sized lunch about an hour ago

E—sudden chest pain while running in the gym

Card 9 PATIENT HISTORY

Dispatch Information: Dispatched to a residence for a patient with chest pain and dyspnea; time is 0200

Scene Size-Up: The patient's wife directs you to the bedroom, where a middle-aged male is experiencing dyspnea; no hazards noted.

Medical History

A—eggs and egg products

M—antibiotics

P—hip replacement 3 weeks ago, bed rest

L—dinner, a sandwich, and a glass of milk

E—awakened from sleep by pain and difficulty breathing

Card 7 CHIEF COMPLAINT

O—gradual onset of confusion, then combativeness

P—hard candy has calmed her somewhat

Q—disoriented to time and place

R—not applicable

S—friends say this is the worst they have seen her

T—slow progression of confusion, then combativeness

AS—alcohol-like odor on breath

PN—none

(Field diagnosis: insulin shock)

Card 8 CHIEF COMPLAINT

O—sudden onset of chest pain

P—deep breathing increases pain

Q—"stabbing"

R—left chest only

S—pain is about 7 on scale of 1 to 10, moderate dyspnea

T—after running, took a deep breath, then started

AS—none

PN—no heart history or irregular pulse

(Field diagnosis: spontaneous pneumothorax)

Card 9 CHIEF COMPLAINT

O—sudden, mild chest pain; patient states, "I can't catch my breath"

P—nothing increases or decreases pain or dyspnea

Q—sharp and stabbing

R—left chest area

S—pain is 4 on a scale of 1 to 10

T—while asleep, sudden and nonprogressive

AS—ashen skin

PN—no dull substernal pain, no history of asthma or chronic obstructive pulmonary disease (COPD)

(Field diagnosis: pulmonary embolism)